Radiant Skin

FROM THE INSIDE OUT

Alan M. Dattner, MD

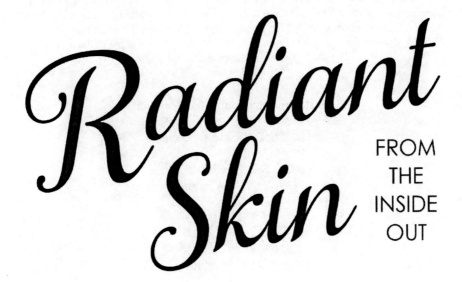

Radiant Skin

FROM THE INSIDE OUT

The Holistic Dermatologist's Guide to Healing Your Skin Naturally

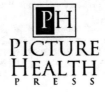

PICTURE HEALTH PRESS

Radiant Skin from the Inside Out:
The Holistic Dermatologist's Guide to Healing Your Skin Naturally

Alan M Dattner, MD
Former Visiting Scientist, Dermatology Branch of National Cancer Institute
Board Certified Dermatologist, Fellow of American Academy of Dermatology (AAD)
Founding member first AAD task force on Nutrition and the Evaluation of Alternative Medicine
Member, Advisory Board for Dermatology: American Botanical Council
Author of the Chapter on Complementary and Alternative Medicine in Dermatology:
Fitzpatrick's *Dermatology in General Medicine*

Illustrations by Ronnie Rae Mendez

HolisticDermatology.com

FIRST EDITION

ISBN: 978-1-942545-16-3
Library of Congress Control Number: 2015946500

Picture Health Press
an Imprint of Wyatt-MacKenzie

Dedication

This book is dedicated to you.
May the natural care of our bodies lead to greater health and beauty
for ourselves and our planet.

Foreword

Recent history has repeatedly witnessed the emergence of new under-standing of the disease process and new healing capabilities, when two medical disciplines are merged together.

Viewing immunology through the lens of biochemistry has led to new frontiers of understanding and therapeutics. Similarly, combining the immunologic technology and understanding with dermatologic illnesses has made dermatology become a rapidly advancing scientific field.

This book describes how Dr. Dattner has combined dermatology with holistic medicine supported by his experience in cellular immunology. He outlines the treatment of dermatologic and inflammatory diseases with this combined approach that he has evolved over the past three decades.

With emphasis on the modification of environmental etiologic factors, Dattner is ushering a new era of possibilities for care of skin diseases — just the beginning of a whole new understanding of diagnostic and treating approaches in dermatology.

Dattner draws from various disciplines that are part of integrative medicine — including nutrition, herbal medicine and other healing modalities. He brings attention to improving digestion and gut microflora, and the integrity of the gut barrier to prevent contents of the digestive tract escaping into the blood and stim-ulating inflammation in the skin. He hones in on likely dietary and environmental sources that may serve as the molecular stimulus to set off a reaction contributing to the disease process.

Applying immunologic principles such as tolerance, and immune cross reactivity, in relation to allergens and organisms from the digestive tract, to clinical care of the skin, Dattner offers a whole host of new possibilities for calming inflammatory skin diseases.

I have known the author since he was a medical student with an interest in immunology, and we both share an interest in dermatology and immunology. Alan Dattner began his immunology research while in college, and continued in his work in several other immunology laboratories before he combined these studies with the skin at the NIH. His interest in emotional factors expanded to an interest in nutritional influences affecting disease and immunity. Over 15 years ago, because of his previous years of experience combining holistic medicine and dermatology, we strongly considered creating the first subdivision of Holistic Dermatology within my dermatology department.

As part of a seminal group of physicians exploring alternative and integrative medicine in the 1980s and 1990s, he was exposed to the evolution and application of nutritional techniques and supplementation to control disease. Alan has combined that understanding with other diagnostic systems such as Applied Kinesiology to try to come to a new understanding of the causal network in dermatologic diseases, and make sense as to what underlying defects are endemic in our society, and how best to treat the individual with a given skin disease.

In this book as in his practice, he puts all the relevant pieces together to try to make sense of what is causing skin disease. The Holistic model used looks across multiple organ systems to restore better balance to those that are most likely to be contributing to the disease process. He illustrates the principles discussed with case reports showing how patients benefited following relevant treatment.

The book is an excellent blueprint for understanding how to combine a variety of natural and conventional methods in treating skin conditions and may prove to be a turning point in the evolution of the Holistic therapy in dermatology.

—Bijan Safai MD, DSc
    Professor & Chairman, Department of Dermatology,
    Professor of Microbiology and Immunology,
    New York Medical College

How to Use This Book

Part One of this book describes some of the underlying issues in the treatment of skin disorders in the organs and processes involved. It will give you the background you need to understand the methods I found effective in natural skincare.

Part Two discusses a number of skin conditions and how to treat them. If you jump ahead to the section most related to the skin problem you have, you may find that you have to return to Part One to get the background understanding you need to get your condition under control.

The preface tells about my medical journey, and how my research and experiences brought me to this knowledge and work.

I've purposely re-stated some information in this book in different ways, both to emphasize its importance, and also to make it convenient to locate when you are reading about treatment of a particular disorder. Another reason for re-stating information is that in reality each condition and set of symptoms, while having important differences, also involves some of the same factors.

Each person develops their condition over a period of time through their own specific exposures with their own genetic uniqueness. So, part of your task in healing is to learn how to undo those issues specific to just you, over a period of time. Part three of this book provides a number of tools to pull together your resources and make the changes necessary to heal. Recognizing the challenge in doing this work, I have made suggestions on how to assemble a team to help you. I have found that making the changes necessary to gain control of skin conditions and inflammation in a natural manner requires extra effort in information-gathering, making changes in diet and lifestyle, and staying on the path long enough to achieve the kind of results you're seeking. Finding and resolving underlying causes can often be a monumental—and satisfying—task, so this book is intended to expand your understanding as you work with your practitioner. People who take this journey in earnest are rewarded doubly with greater self-awareness and improvements in vitality, energy, and health.

TABLE OF CONTENTS

Part 1

HOLISTIC MEDICINE, YOUR SKIN, AND YOUR HEALTH

Part 2

SKIN AND SKIN CONDITIONS

Part 3

PREPARING FOR YOUR HOLISTIC EXPERIENCE

Preface: My Story

What a strange combination: holistic and dermatology! Unlike internal medicine, routine dermatology is often practiced as if it were dealing with only one organ, at the most superficial level of the body. We often think of simply putting something *on the skin,* rather than inside the body. So it's somewhat of a paradox to consider treating the skin by treating the rest of the body.

How did I become one of the first dermatologists to declare this as a specialty? What were the motivations and learning experiences that brought me the expertise needed? I would like to share with you the pathway of my life that led me to this unique and eclectic approach. There is no way I could have planned this journey at its onset more than six decades ago. When I began my training 40 years ago, holistic dermatology didn't exist. There was and is no instruction manual or course series taught in medical school or dermatologic residency, on treating the skin holistically.

As a child I had many illnesses, but was passionately interested in science, for which I was ostracized by others in my classes. Getting used to accept thinking differently became important in following my own insights from research, study, and experience, which frequently contradicted the dogma held by the majority of my peers.

One summer during college, I got a volunteer position in a small lab at a research facility in Rye, NY called Sloane Kettering. Most of the facility was devoted to putting every sort of stuff imaginable into cancer cell cultures to see what would be useful in killing cancer. But this particular lab, under Dr. Lloyd Old (sometimes referred to as the father of tumor immunology for the many things he did and discovered in his career) was focused on tumor immunology. I began reading the literature and observing the studies on the subject.

I was accepted to medical school after three years of college. At NYU Medical School we had an unusually large number of incredible immunologists in various departments, and in addition to my coursework, I was able to attend many thought-provoking lectures. But my interest always wandered beyond learning what was already known in medicine, so I spent time in a lab that was doing experimental work in kidney transplantation, skin grafting, and correlating the transplantation antigen system in humans.

I felt compelled to do further studies in cellular immunology, so I joined the honors program, which allowed me to take time off from my clinical studies and do research. Ironically, although I was at a school with numerous renowned immunologists, the most exciting lab to me was not at NYU, but rather at the Albert Einstein College of Medicine. I chose to work with Dr. Barry R. Bloom, who guided me to study one of the first substances that allowed communication between two types of white blood cells in the immune system; lymphocytes and macrophages.

Dr. Bloom turned out to be a great mentor and an outstanding visionary scientist, as he later was chosen to head the Harvard School of Public Health for several years.

In the late 1960s I went to Northern California and experienced California culture, and a whole new way of looking at the influence of other realms including diet, emotions, and spirit on health. I began to see that an entire world of relevant factors were being left out of my otherwise excellent medical education. My early experiences with illness, what I was discovering in the laboratory, and what I saw in California, deepened my curiosity about the effects of emotions on immunity and illness. I went to San Francisco General Hospital for my internship, and was exposed to intensive medicine training, and more of the California philosophy about healing. When I finished, I traveled back across the country and met some of the important figures in the world of psychosomatic research at the University of Rochester and Stanford University Medical Center.

Following that I went to New York to a dermatology residency at Albert Einstein College of medicine, started by a colleague of mine and spent my last two years there doing immunology research half-time in two different laboratories. One of the papers that came out of our work in 1974 was one of the first on Kaposi's sarcoma and immunosuppression, and turned out to be one of the first on what was later called AIDS. I did a study on psychological stress and *in vitro* immune reactivity in breast cancer patients. Next, I worked with Dr. Arye Rubenstein studying lymphocyte receptors in synchronized lymphoma cells.

I wanted to continue my studies on the immune system as well as dermatology, so I located someone at the dermatology branch of the National Cancer Institute who was doing that kind of research. Between my chief, Dr. William R.

Levis and me, we had over 25 years of experience in cellular immunology and dermatology, perhaps more than any other dermatologist-immunologist team in the world at that time. The main thrust of our work was identifying the nature of recognition of foreign substances by lymphocytes in a delayed hypersensitivity system. We basically demonstrated that lymphocytes recognize not only the foreign substance, or antigen, but also recognized the *histocompatibility* complex of the white blood cells presenting that antigen. The work we did was similar to the work of two later Nobel Prizes in Medicine in 1980 and 1996. We began to understand the nature of what is now known as cross-reactive immune recognition, or molecular mimicry. Once we had demonstrated the concept of cross-reactivity in a human cellular immune assay, I began to understand that inflammation in skin disease was likely to be caused by a very specific cross-reactive response in patients. From this I could understand how *very different foods, infections, or chemical exposures* could lead to a particular inflammatory skin condition in different individuals. Something profound occurred to me: the cause of an inflammatory reaction in skin disease is a similarity between an aggravating substance and some target on that person's skin. It is not a specific substance that causes each disease, but rather an equation of similarity between trigger and target for that specific individual that sets off the disease process.

I looked, but there was no academic institution where I could continue studies on immunity skin disease and nutrition, so I joined one of the first holistic clinics in the Northeast of the country, Integral Health Services, an offshoot of the Integral Yoga Institute. There we included the interaction of nutrition and many other healing disciplines in treating patients. The community and the local hospital also needed a dermatologist, so I became the community dermatologist and gradually merged my holistic treatments with my general practice of dermatology.

Along the way I joined a seminal group of holistic physicians in the Northeast, and attended integrative medicine conferences and herbal conferences. I learned herbology and Applied Kinesiology. Regular attendance of herbal, Complementary and Alternative Medicine, and integrative medical conferences, has built my knowledge. For the 25 years, I've been presenting speeches at Integrative and Dermatologic conferences, writing articles for the professional journals, reviewing professional articles on nutrition and dermatology, testing and evaluating products, supplying answers to popular magazines on holistic dermatology and the skin, and of course, seeing thousands of patients. All of this has contributed to my deeper understanding of the effects of holistic measures on the skin, and reflected on my experience in these matters.

I became involved as a founding member of the American Academy of Dermatology's Task Force on Nutrition and the Evaluation of Alternative Medicine and have presented nationally and internationally on my work and experience.

For the past 14 years I have restricted my practice to Holistic Dermatology and Integrative Medicine. At this point in my career I want to share what I have learned with my colleagues and the rest of the world. Fostering the application of the insights I have developed and want the world to experience has become my passion. It is time to expand my unique system of tailoring choices for diagnosis and treatment of it inflammatory skin and other diseases using an integrative and holistic model. I hope that this book expands the diagnostic and therapeutic tools that dermatologists have to help their patients, just as the growing worlds of pharmaceuticals and lasers and other modalities are doing.

As the condition of the skin is related to what is going on inside the body, so too the condition of both is related to the environmental condition of that very important interface we live on, the "Skin of the Earth." I suggested to a past president of the American Academy of Dermatology to have our organization consider this topic as a contribution to world health, just as we lobby for sun protection and early detection of skin cancers, as a public health service. This never quite got off the ground, so I have devoted a chapter to this in the book. I offer this perspective to you, as you and your children can only be as healthy as the toxins in your environment allow.

Introduction

How do you clear your skin problem and make your skin more beautiful using natural methods? What methods address the physiology understood by dermatologists, but make your skin more beautiful by placing a much greater emphasis on nutrition and supplements to rebalance your underlying condition? I have spent over three decades developing an answer to that question based on my immunology research and the emerging science behind Functional and Integrative Medicine and many other healing disciplines. I share that understanding in this book so that you can find help in making interpretations of your exposures, and treatment responses to guide you through a multi-systems approach to healing your skin with an emphasis on natural methods.

Seekers may be confused by the vast array of advertised products, systems, alternative practitioners, products, and testimonials found on the Internet claiming success with improving the disease you believe you have. From my perspective, you acquired your skin disease by your own very unique path, and need to identify and account for that path in order to make the right choices in a real and ongoing way to truly improve your condition. It took many years to develop your condition so you should consider spending at least that many months of lifestyle change to improve it. This book outlines my working understanding of how the various systems of the body and the environment interact to make your condition better or worse, so that you can better understand the context in which a treatment or diet was reported to work, and understand whether it is relevant to you.

When you read stories of amazing cures by various practitioners, product salespeople, and individuals cured of a particular disease, you will know how to decide if those stories might be helpful to you. It can be easy to get carried away with a treatment program that was specific to *someone else* whose condition has the same name as yours, even though your condition is in fact *unique to you*. Because of this plethora of conflicting voices, each patient now needs a basic understanding of immunology and digestive physiology in order to determine what makes most sense for a personal, particular condition.

There are many miracles of modern medicine, for both diagnosis and treatment of skin disease. And there are many other traditions of healing that embody knowledge gained back through millennia, which are the foundation for complementary medicine techniques we know today. Where one path alone is not always effective, a combination of paths yields the potential to obtain the best results. That's where this book comes in.

My intention is to ground you in an understanding of the body's workings that underlie inflammation and skin disease, so that you will have a sound foundation from which to make choices among the vast therapeutic options available. I'm honored to share what I've learned over the past four decades as a dermatologist who has an extensive background in immunology, having used a variety of nutritional, herbal, and other alternative approaches to treating skin disorders.

In many cases, skin disorders are *symptoms* of underlying problems. You will begin learning to unravel the variety of issues that lead to inflammation of your skin. Understanding basic principles of how the immune system works will help you to better navigate the myriad of overlapping concepts necessary to choose what you eat and what treatments you employ to heal your skin. These same principles also apply to inflammation elsewhere in the body, and to autoimmune diseases as well.

This book will help you identify those practitioners who can help you best. It is not meant to diagnose, prevent, or treat disease. A good practitioner has a breadth of experience and knowledge and also helps you see and address your blind spots: the thoughts or activities contributing to your illness that you somehow just cannot see. It would be impossible in one book to share all of what I know about the conditions discussed.

I have written this book primarily for patients and the general public, omitting much of the technical details and supportive references that would be in a scientific treatise or a course for physicians. It does offer physicians an overview of methods to control skin diseases naturally.

We'll start with some basic principles that are vital to understanding this work, and then discuss specific conditions. The patient stories are based on actual people (whose names and identifying details have been changed). The first section of the book explains some of the principles you need to know to understand the holistic approach and how different systems of the body are involved. The second section focuses on specific skin diseases. The last section gives you tools to gather information, and make the changes that are necessary to improve your underlying health naturally.

This book is my gift to the world, derived from the knowledge and love given to me from all of my teachers, colleagues, and patients.

Part 1

HOLISTIC MEDICINE, YOUR SKIN, AND YOUR HEALTH

CHAPTER 1

WHAT IS HOLISTIC MEDICINE?

Pushing Beyond Limits

I am passionate about pushing beyond the limits of conventional medical wisdom in finding solutions to patients' medical problems. I am captivated by the vast sea of chronic illnesses that defies cure, that condemns people to suffer and dwindle away to the anguish of their friends and loved ones, and that leaves people and their physicians and caregivers with a frustrating sense of futility. Stories of miraculous successes, alternative cures, and spontaneous healing only further fuel my desire to find solutions where none exist, especially when so many physicians offer nothing more than relief of symptoms. I want to share the insights I have gained in evolving a system for treating skin disease in a more natural way, so that others can gain perspective on how the pieces of such a program work together. I want my readers to see how various diet changes and treatments are applied according to the individual as well as the condition, and work in the hands of a board certified dermatologist who is grounded in study of the immune system.

I recently read an article where two major experts in dermatology (whom I respect for many reasons) were quoted as saying that that we don't have enough information yet to say whether diet affects acne. From my point of view, we may or may not be able to find the kind of scientific proof these experts are seeking, but as I go about what I do every day and make people better, it makes it awfully hard for me to deny that diet affects acne (and the most recent medical literature is beginning to agree with what I've found). Some of the things I recommend to my patients may not be part of the medical establishment's standard treatments. But I know they work—and so do my patients.

I see pathways to healing through a web of information that I have watched grow richer and more tangible over half a century. This informational tapestry has grown both more complex and better understood as the piercing eye of science and the wisdom of ancient insight have cast increasing light on the inner workings of our being.

I personally have watched the growth of cellular immunology, from my summer volunteering with Dr. Lloyd Old, the founder of tumor immunology, through reading the work of the early giants of the field, to meeting and working with those of my generation, and to making my own palpable contributions to the field three decades ago. I was part of the early movement toward holistic medicine. In 1973, my boyhood friend, Michael Samuels, wrote *The Well Body Book* and a series of the first holistic medical books written by a physician. And I had the privilege of a first-rate medical education and residency in some of the finest centers in one of the greatest cities in the world, New York. Along the way, I have learned from thousands of professors, teachers, colleagues, patients, and healers.

I have had added each experience to my own mental tapestry of How It All Works. Sometimes confirming, sometimes enlarging, sometimes modifying, sometimes changing, each experience is a footnote to the personal truth of my vision. This vision has helped me see ahead by decades the future for the world of medicine and healing. Though such vision is never twenty-twenty, it has equipped me with the insight to help people with options they never had before, and for that I am very grateful. It has also helped me align with and see what is coming, often well before the products I am using emerge in the mainstream marketplace.

After years of being ridiculed for the path and interest I took toward my dermatology and medicine, I find myself right in the middle of a great fascination with natural and dietary approaches to healing skin problems and making the skin beautiful which has caught up to my own work. I seek to make a real difference in health and the transformation of the predominant working models used for healing. I have been fortunate enough to be quoted in many different kinds of publications, and I am now being sought after as an expert in the world of natural skin and beauty treatment. Unfortunately, because of time and space constraints, I haven't been able to say as much as I'd like to about these topics, or fully express my passion for my chosen field. It's finally time to speak about how these streams of holistic philosophy are interrelated, and how you can use these ideas to improve your health. I am happy to finally be able to share things about how health works that I was unable to share in the past.

The natural treatment methods I have developed over several decades are having good results with those people who follow them and I want to let the world know about them. **Above all, I want those who suffer from inflammatory skin diseases, and their physicians, to know that there are other, more natural ways to get inflammatory skin diseases, and indeed *any* inflammatory conditions, under control. This book explains how it is done, and why it works.**

So What is Holistic Dermatology?

When you come to a dermatologist with a skin condition, you want to know what it is and what the dermatologist can give you to make it go away. You may also be curious about what caused it, why you got it then, and why you got it where you did. You hope that there is one clear diagnosis and one basic prescription that you can take or apply to make it go away. Conventional dermatology is all you need if your experience goes that way. If the problem keeps coming back again and again, if there are a lot of other problems going on with your digestion and other systems that you sense may be associated with your skin, then you need holistic dermatology. If you have side effects from conventional treatments, want the safest treatments to be tried first, or are concerned about the short or long term side effects of ingredients in your skin medications, you need a holistic treatment. If you have been trying one thing after another with minimal lasting results, you need an additional diagnosis of the underlying array of causes going on *in you*. If your patterns leading to your dermatitis, such as unhealthy eating, are stuffing an emotional hole you dare not peer into, you need to commit yourself to a holistic approach to fixing your skin. Holistic care requires you to take responsibility for your actions and be an active participant in the healing process.

One of the first questions I get from people upon hearing that I practice Holistic Dermatology is, "What do you do in Holistic Dermatology that is different from regular dermatology?" Holistic dermatology is the name I gave to the type of dermatology I practiced when I joined a holistic medical clinic associated with the Integral Yoga Institute in 1979. Over the years, my work truly became more holistic. Holistic refers to treating the totality of the patient: medical, physical, emotional, and even spiritual, as needed. It also implies being eclectic—using not only good medicine, but looking to the latest science and applying it, as well as using tools from other healing modalities, such as nutrition, herbal medicine, applied kinesiology, and aspects of Ayurveda, Chinese medicine, and other systems. Combining these tools is done individually according to the particular skills of the practitioner and the needs of the patient.

For many patients, holistic medicine also refers to applying natural and safer methods before resorting to drugs or surgery, being vegan or vegetarian, and being environmentally conscious of the surface of the earth on which we live (later chapters will cover this subject).

In short, I treat the underlying cause(s) of a patient's skin condition. I treat the causal factors that aggravate the specific individual I am seeing. My prescription focuses more on diet, nutritional supplements, and herbs than on drugs and surgery, but I use western modalities when they are the best option for the situation. For example, the inflammation in acne or eczema is treated by identifying and removing the cause. If food aggravators are discovered, the food is eliminated and digestive function is improved with herbs and supplements so that the allergens from the foods do not get out into the target tissues. I then use supplements and herbs to help get rid of the aggravating allergens or toxins by enhancing the function of organs of excretion including the kidneys, liver, intestines, lymphatics, and lungs. I avoid antibiotics except when absolutely necessary. I rebalance hormones using natural herbs and supplements rather than birth control pills. This is very different from the conventional method of applying and administering immunosuppressants (drugs that dampen down the activity of the immune system) as the main way to control an inflammatory condition.

Because dermatologists normally deal with diseases of the skin, many people think that I deal with surface issues. But the truth is I look at patients' insides to find out the cause of what is happening on the outside. Since foods, chemicals, infections, and stress often lead to inflammation, and inflammation is the process that causes allergy, autoimmunity, and many of the diseases of the skin, my burning passion is to identify whatever it is that provoked the immune system to start its virulent attack in the first place. That's what inflammation is—an attack by white blood cells, antibodies, and other immune system chemicals at the site of an irritation, injury, or infection. These chemicals and blood cells have good intentions; they are actually there to facilitate healing. But as with too much of any good thing, they often end up causing heat, redness, swelling, pain, and sometimes loss of function. It is our body's defense system gone awry. And unfortunately, inflammation has been found to play a significant role not only in dermatological conditions, but in common health issues such diabetes, heart disease, allergies, asthma, and arthritis, to name just a few.

I strongly believe that, rather than repeatedly using steroid creams and immunosuppressants for weeks, months, or years, the wiser course is to figure out what is likely to be causing the problem and treat it with gentler, more natural means. Conventional dermatologists often inquire about what was going on just before the skin condition began. I ask questions to find out what set the stage for the patient's immune and other organ systems to permit such a reaction in the first place. This may include searching for chronic hidden infection and environmental sensitivity and toxicity. I also look for emotional conflicts that eat up the individual's health from the inside out.

Ginny's Acne

Ginny's acne was so bad that she needed two separate courses of Accutane (a powerful vitamin A derivative) to get it under control over the course of two years, during her later teens. Antibiotics and topical medications kept it under control, but it slowly came back when she stopped using these medications. She became more health conscious, and came to me for a more natural form of treatment. The numerous pimples of her lower face began clearing on the diet and supplements, and she began feeling better as well, including loss of weight and resolution of her constipation alternating with diarrhea. An unexpected benefit of my program was improvement of chronic joint pain that woke her up at night from time to time.

Lapses off the diet, such as wine at her best friend's wedding, were followed by temporary outbreaks. Over time, Ginny stopped the supplements and went back to her former diet, which included lots of sugar, simple carbohydrates, and some beer and wine, and her acne and other symptoms slowly returned. She got back on the program again, and after a month of diet and supplements, her acne and digestive issues improved, and her joint pains and energy began to improve. This story illustrates that for Ginny and many other people, acne is part of a more fundamental issue related to food and the digestive system, and that correcting the problem also improves inflammation in other parts of the body.

Why Go Holistic?

Why not just go to your local dermatologist and get the latest conventional treatments for your skin disorder? These treatments are scientifically approved and paid for by your insurance. They often involve the latest and most sophisticated chemical drugs, which have gone through millions of dollars' worth of testing and have been approved by the FDA after a rigorous process. And, it might not be a bad idea to get the expertise in skin diagnosis, for dermatologists excel in that form of categorization. If you have a puzzling or difficult skin condition, a dermatologist is one of the first physicians you should see. Their expertise in diagnosis of skin conditions, whether or not you use the treatment they recommend, will give you a valuable perspective on what is going on and what the causes may be. Perhaps you have an acute problem that clears completely with treatment. That's a good thing. But some people who respond initially to conventional treatments find that their condition returns again and again and that they need stronger medication each time to suppress and control it. Other people don't improve at all. Sometimes a skin rash will clear completely through conventional treatment, but not removing the underlying problem serves only to drive the actual issue deeper underground. For example, giving oral steroids for inflammation resulting from a chronic infection weakens the immune systems and may allow that infection to spread.

When suppressive pharmaceuticals are prescribed, they rarely address the conditions that lead to chronic disease in the first place, such as environmental exposure to allergens. And unfortunately there is a chance that the side effects of pharmaceuticals will dangerously outweigh the benefits they confer. Topical steroids can stop an itch that prevents sleep or leads to scratching and infection, but chronic use of topical steroids can lead to infection, thin the skin permanently, and may even suppress the adrenal glands. Oral steroids and more potent immunosuppressants can stop a dangerous allergic or inflammatory reaction that threatens life or function. Unfortunately, they can also paralyze the immune system so that dangerous infections such as tuberculosis can take hold, or tumors such as lymphoma can start to grow. Many patients who are not helped by current therapeutic paradigms are beginning to question what they are being told by the medical and pharmaceutical establishment, by insurance companies, and by the government agencies that oversee our collective health care.

The first problem is that we are beginning to recognize that each person with a given skin condition has his or her own individual circumstance that contributes to developing that disorder. The concept of "disease" made it much more possible to classify and treat disorders. But the idea of every person with the same disease needing to be treated in exactly the same way breaks down in face of knowledge of human genetic individuality, epigenetic changes (see box below), environmental exposures, individual life experiences, and the perspective of various folk healing systems Our current insurance payment system is also based on the small bag of tricks to make symptoms go away. It is almost impossible for a well-trained professional to take the time to get a detailed history, diagnose and treat the imbalances in multiple systems, and transmit all the new information to change a patient's diet and lifestyle within the reimbursement paid for under insurance.

What We Mean When We Talk About "Disease"

The whole concept of disease is a kind of simplification of a lot of different signs, symptoms, lab tests results, genetic traits, and other findings that we lump together for ease of understanding what is occurring in someone. My colleague and mentor, Dr. Sid Baker, once said that people often think of a disease as "something that jumped out from behind a tree and grabbed you as if it was an actual entity." According to that thinking, everyone with the same disease is grabbed by the same entity, so everyone with any given skin condition needs the same treatment.

If that were true, a given course of treatment that was successful in one person should be successful in another. *Most of the studies on diseases are performed as if this is so.* For all the brilliance and advances medical science has brought, it still suffers from the basic flaw in thinking that people with the same condition always come from the same causes and therefore must need the same treatment. So, various treatments are used to see if they make a disease go away in a big enough percentage of people with a given disease. If a given treatment works in just a few people, it is assumed to be coincidence, and the treatment is declared a failure. Under the assumption that everyone with the same disease is the same, success of a treatment in only a sub-set of a treatment trial is dismissed as statistically insignificant, even though it may really be working in that sub-set of the group.

Why is this an error in thinking? First, in good dermatology and medicine, we recognize and look for distinctions of cause in many cases. And we now know that there are a lot of genetic variants that are responsible for both similar and different defects in biochemical reactions, even leading to the same disease. A disease develops as a consequence of a concert of factors. This stage is set by a genetic tendency to form the reaction characteristic of the disease.

The concept of a disease has helped us greatly in classifying skin and medical conditions, but it breaks down when we assume that everyone got to that disease by a similar set of causes. We now know a disease comes about on account of genetic and environmental exposures, so that not everybody gets the same disease in the same way. Why medicine clings so tightly to the disease theory in the face of this information, as if knowing the disease will tell you the treatment to get rid of it, is baffling in the context of this information on individual genetic specificity.

What's more, people have specific genes that are "open" and others that are "shut down," according to conditions in their life. So, conditions that activate a given gene could make your "waffle iron" (template for making proteins) open to make its protein waffles, while your twin brother, who has lived in different conditions, has his similar genetic waffle iron closed. The latest information is that our genetic expression actually gets modified in response to environmental exposures in what is known as an "epigenetic" process ("epigenetic" refers to external modifications to DNA that turn genes "on" or "off." These modifications do not change the DNA sequence, but instead, they affect how cells "read" genes).

What's the Matter with Conventional Dermatology?

Millions of people with all kinds of skin problems are helped by conventional dermatology, including diagnosing and treating acute conditions, contact dermatitis, diagnosis and removal of cancers, reduction of aging effects, identification of underlying systemic diseases, and a variety of other problems. It is based on the latest science. So why should you want to look to holistic dermatology? One problem is the chance of getting swept up in side effects. Another problem is that a number of people slip through the cracks of the system and find themselves with chronic skin problems that don't seem to go away. Some even find that they have a number of other health issues that continue to get worse even though they are told those problems are unrelated to their skin. Some people find themselves so messed up from their conditions and the problems that came after the treatments that they cannot lead normal lives. Many of the treatments used in conventional dermatology are aimed at blocking the symptoms rather than fixing the underlying problem.

I recently read an article on a newly discovered mechanism related to inflammation, followed by the statement that this would give us new opportunities to block this mechanism, thus stopping the inflammation from progressing. Blocking makes a lot of sense when stopping a process will prevent irreversible harm, improve your appearance, relieve immediate anxiety, or help in a situation where deeper change is not possible. It makes less sense in a chronic disorder, when it is possible to discover and correct whatever is provoking the situation. Current pharmacology is based on blocking the mechanisms discovered, and the premise that we cannot discover and alter the cause. Holistic treatment uses the same science, but is based on discovering what is provoking the inflammation, and removing the provocation and the conditions that allow it to happen. When the provocation can be removed, other issues resolve, the chronic condition calms down, and the collateral damage from throwing a monkey wrench into the body's physiologic machinery does not occur. It is always worth trying if the individual is motivated, willing, and able.

Modern dermatology just does not work hard enough at finding and correcting underlying causes if the problem persists. And patients are not expected to make lifestyle changes frequently enough to make uncovering these corrections possible. For example, corticosteroids applied topically or taken systemically often calm down the inflammation; however, the inflammation frequently comes back when these drugs are stopped.

In the case of corticosteroids, there is a progressive loss of effectiveness over time so that it becomes necessary to use stronger and stronger versions to get the same effect. Prolonged use of stronger corticosteroids causes thinning of the skin so that the blood vessels show through and the skin becomes shiny with loss of normal protective characteristics. This is especially true on the face, where some people can be damaged permanently by as little as a month's application of more potent topical corticosteroids. Steroid acne can also occur, and this is extremely hard to get under control without the use of more drugs. Because corticosteroids suppress the immune system, the patient is at greater risk for bacterial and fungal infections.

Another major problem from using suppressive therapy such as topical corticosteroids and the whole issue of treating the skin as an isolated organ unrelated to the rest of the body is that underlying problems, reflected in the skin, are missed earlier in their progression when they would be easier to resolve. The skin is a window reflecting what is going on inside the body. Conventional dermatology does an excellent job in teaching dermatologists how to spot rare and life-threatening conditions by examining the skin. For example, some patients with abnormally stretchy skin resulting from a condition known as Ehlers-Danlos Syndrome have problems with not only the elastin of their skin, but also the elastin in their blood vessels. As a result, when this condition is diagnosed, the patient may be referred to a specialist for evaluation of their blood vessels and the potential risk of a major blood vessel rupturing, leading to internal bleeding and death. Unfortunately, much less training is provided to recognize common conditions that involve such issues as digestion and food allergy. As a result, many dermatologists fail to alert their patients that their skin condition may be related to what they eat, so the patient continues to aggravate their inner issues while they suppress the outward signs with drugs.

You know how disturbing it is to be driving your car and see one of the dashboard warning lights come on. It might tell you that there are problems with oil, battery, overheating, or general engine issues. The alert can be triggered by something simple that is easily checked and corrected, or it could be an indication that you're headed for disaster if you do not investigate. Imagine putting black tape over the warning lights so that you wouldn't need to look at them. For some people, suppressing the symptoms on the skin is a little like blacking out the flashing warning lights on your dashboard. So another problem with suppressive therapy, especially prolonged suppressive therapy, is that you missed the opportunity to deal with a warning and correct the underlying problem early on, before significant damage is done. You allow the underlying disorders to fester and create more problems that you will then have to deal with later.

Risk of significant damaging side effects is another problem with the use of conventional medications for treating skin diseases. You may decide to take that risk when the threat from the skin condition itself is sufficient. Or, if the appearance of your skin condition is severe, it may make sense for you to take a powerful internal medication. Many people can tolerate oral and injected forms of cortisone without significant problem. But it's important to know that the side effects can include serious infections and cancers, psychosis, precipitation of diabetes, damage to the digestive tract, and a host of other health risks.

Other drugs that suppress the immune system were designed to create less collateral damage. One such drug, known as Raptiva, was taken off the market because of its dangerous side effects. So the problem with the more potent drugs that stop inflammation is not necessarily that they will cause severe damage, but that they have a potential for doing so.

Another problem with using drugs on a chronic basis to treat acne is that they can cause problems that require compensations by the body, requiring more drugs to correct those issues. For instance, antibiotics destroy some of the normal bacteria in our intestines, only to allow them to be replaced by overgrowth of other types of bacteria that are resistant to those antibiotics, or yeast.. The delicate balance among the hundred trillion or so microorganisms that inhabit our large intestines gets thrown off by antibiotics, causing progressive subtle disturbances that may take years to identify and correct. A variety of side effects from this, including yeast overgrowth, leakage of food allergens into the bloodstream, digestive issues, and inflammation of the skin and other tissues of the body can result. This book discusses these issues and how to treat them.

To be fair, many dermatologists have insights into specific natural treatments, but they are not equipped to address skin conditions through a predominantly natural approach in most cases. They usually do not have the training and experience. And under the shrinking insurance reimbursement and rising expenses and government requirements from various agencies, they do not have the time to probe into the network of experiences that caused a given patient to develop their skin condition. Nor do they have the staff and tools to inform and motivate patients about the many changes they need to make.

It is likely that the majority of people with skin disorders will continue to use medications to control their conditions. The challenge of following diets, costs beyond what insurance covers, lack of availability of doctors who understand both the skin and nutritional medicine, and difficulty in finding out what is in our food and environment are all factors that make suppressive therapy the practical solution. For those who fail such therapy, or are motivated to correct the cause in a safer manner, holistic treatment makes sense.

How Holistic Dermatology Can Help

Instead of simply suppressing the reaction in the skin, holistic dermatology seeks to correct the cause and remove it so that healing can occur. Sometimes causes have to be removed in the same manner as peeling layers of an onion. Removal of food allergens and allergens from the environment, fixing the digestive system, and enhancing the body's ability to break down and eliminate allergic and toxic products are the major tools used. Government regulations, standards of practice, and requirements for proof of efficacy of treatments have whittled down drug treatments to a relatively limited number of options. Nature has provided a much broader number of remedies, many of which have been discovered and used over the past thousands of years. Traditions passed down over the centuries provide guidelines for their use among the spectrum of choices available to an individual for treating their disorder. Often there are emotional and psychological issues deeply entwined with the factors that initiate the skin condition. In some cases, these issues need to be confronted and resolved to allow a more complete healing. This book is a blueprint for how to correct the inner conditions that lead to inflammatory skin disorders, and indeed, to all sorts of inflammatory conditions of the body.

Holistic Medicine's Gains in the Past 50 Years

While people in Germany and France have been using homeopathic medicine for the past hundred years and consider it normal (one out of three drugs prescribed in Germany is an herb), this country has taken much longer to return to the roots of natural and holistic medicine.

Early in my medical career, I had to keep my practice of complementary methods very quiet. Letting people know was dangerous. Speaking up about my work at medical meetings in the 1970s, 80s, and into the 90s, I was sharply criticized and threatened by other physicians who towed the line of conventional medicine. But over the past two decades, there has been a very powerful sea change in what patients are demanding and what practitioners are providing. Patients want answers that make more sense. Let's take a look at some signs of this sea change.

In a report from the National Health Institute, a nationwide government survey from December 2008 stated that approximately 38 percent of U.S. adults aged 18 years and over, and approximately 12 percent of children, used some form of Complementary and Alternative Medicine (CAM). And almost half the adults between ages 50-59 used some form of CAM.

The World Health Organization estimates that between 65 to 80 percent of the world's population (about 3 billion people) rely on what we call alternative medicine as their primary form of health care.

In 1998, the American Medical Association (AMA) introduced Resolution 514, "encouraging its members to become better informed regarding alternative medicine and to participate in appropriate studies of it." Almost one-third of American medical schools—among them Harvard, Yale, Johns Hopkins, and Georgetown Universities—now offer coursework in alternative methods.

The American Holistic Medical Association (AHMA) was founded in 1978 to unite licensed physicians who practice holistic medicine. It is the oldest holistic medicine organization of its kind, and many of today's national leaders in holistic medicine got their start as members of the AHMA. Today, there are numerous organizations dedicated to holistic and integrative medical care, under an ever-growing list of titles.

Diagnosis and Treatment, Holistically Speaking

In this chapter, I have discussed a variety of factors that account for health in a holistic model. I would like to summarize the essence of how they bring me to a level of decision-making for diagnosis and treatment that you probably won't find in a traditional medical approach. I must emphasize that nearly every principle I describe in this book is supported by good science or someone's good practice. It's just that I put them together in a package approach that is not commonly found in my specialty of dermatology or in conventional medicine.

Diagnostically, I include the conventional medical diagnosis as an important starting point, but by no means the final definition of the patient's ailment. I look for what caused the problem to develop in that specific individual. I look for genetic and environmental factors that would cause the expression of the genes involved, as well as for resultant body compensation for the problems. I consider carefully a whole host of factors that come with living in our culture in America and factors of the sub-culture in which one lives as well. Those cultural factors define many of the environmental challenges to which we are subjected. High sugar, high yeast, high stress, fast eating, poor digestion, hormonal dis-regulation, unbalanced fatty acid, and over-nutrition are pretty common problems for people in this culture. Just by looking at a patient and asking a few questions, I can confirm or dispute this initial set of expectations.

I weigh many different forms of evidence and make my own well-educated decisions, while my academic and legal colleagues await official proof from multiple randomly controlled double-blind investigations. I have begun to trust the combination of personal experience, animal and in vitro laboratory data, anecdotal and suggestive reports in the medical and lay literature, and information from other healing disciplines such as acupuncture, Ayurveda, homeopathy, and functional medicine. I reach my diagnosis when a number of these different information sources align with my experience and what is plausible or likely from my investigation of the cutting edge data in the scientific literature.

This, of course, is done in conjunction with getting a careful history from that individual of all the events that led up to the onset of the rash or illness in question. Indeed, I make my patient a deputy detective in sleuthing the hidden cause. This is one of the most important sources I have to explain the root of the illness. I educate my patient to comb his or her history for exposures or events that could contribute, according to the type of environmental triggers I might expect.

I examine information that I was taught to dismiss as irrelevant during my training, during which we were told that there were numerous inflammatory conditions with unknown causes, and these were to be treated with corticosteroids and anti-inflammatories to calm down the symptoms.

I also bring other healing disciplines into my work that may or may not coincide with the medical theory. I include the perspective of Psychosomatic Medicine, Functional Medicine, and with my assistants, of Ayurvedic medicine. I use a form of muscle response testing known as Applied Kinesiology to help refine my diagnoses and choices. I am open to getting additional help from whatever perspective is reasonable and available.

In a way, my method involves going "out on a limb" to make a diagnosis and choose treatment. Fortunately, that limb is supported by an array of what my colleagues would consider "soft data": not enough to constitute a proof, but more than enough to make you look harder at the possible relationship. So I move forward and further out toward my treatment strategy, supported by many beams of soft data bolstering my conclusions from below and suspending them from above. One of those suspensions is the knowledge that tens of thousands of alternative practitioners use some form of the treatments and diagnostic tests that I am employing, with apparent success, in related conditions. I am comforted on my suspended perch, knowing full well the superior risk and benefit profile of taking holistic as apposed to the conventional path to treatment. I share the considerations for that choice with my patients, many of whom are in the medical field themselves and have chosen to join me on that very well-supported limb.

Summary
What's Different about Holistic Dermatology?

Conventional dermatology and holistic dermatology share many of the same goals. They both strive to help you fix your problem skin and improve your outward appearance. Holistic dermatology, however, has more of an emphasis on healing from many different perspectives and from the inside out so that you are eliminating the underlying causes and not just the symptoms.

It is eclectic and strong in many different disciplines; it requires individual responsibility from the patient; and it strives to find and treat the deeper layers of cause rather than focusing on blocking the inflammatory process. You will find out more about the inner workings of holistic dermatology and its healing powers as you continue to read this book. The appropriate combination of Holistic therapies with current treatment offers a new level of effectiveness for the population with chronic and recalcitrant dermatologic disorders.

CHAPTER 2

THE VALUE OF INSIGHT AND INTUITION IN MEDICINE

A major component of holistic medicine is using information that makes sense from the totality of evidence surrounding a situation, but before it is "officially" known or proven. For example, decades before the official notification was issued, many holistic practitioners were warning patients about the dangers of smoking, of trans-saturated fatty acids, and of high-fructose corn syrup-containing soft drinks.

Before a piece of information becomes popular knowledge, or even knowledge to oneself, it is often intuitively known. In my physical chemistry course, I learned that some of the most important proofs came intuitively first and then scientists spent many years or even a lifetime proving them. After years of studying carbon bonds, the nineteenth century organic chemist, Kekulé, in trying to figure out the structure of the organic chemical, benzene, went into a reverie in front of a fire and saw snakes chasing their tales. From that he realized that benzene had a circular ring structure, which he later showed to be so. In his book *Blink*, author Malcom Gladwell talks about "the power of thinking without thinking," which means knowing or believing something on a gut or instinctual level before there is actual proof. I believe that many people can have insights into what will develop in the future in their area of expertise. For example, thirty years ago, many technologists predicted how the Internet would unfold as it is today.

In the field of medicine more than thirty years ago, I was conducting studies on immunology at the NIH, and intuitively understood ways in which this knowledge could eventually be used. It has been amazing to look at what I was learning then and the fact that I was able to predict how it would develop decades later (I will discuss some examples of my insights and how they pertain to the treatments suggested in later chapters as a way to demonstrate the validity of my ideas about the future of medicine).

How Do You "Know" What You Know?

When I use the terms "knowing" and pre-knowing," I am not talking about anything magical or psychic in nature. I am, after all, a doctor, not an illusionist. There is a kind of knowing that comes from immersing yourself in as much information as possible about a subject from every angle. In holistic medicine, trustworthy health methods are woven from clinical observation of different schools of healing techniques, scientific data, epidemiologic data, and observed results. Diagnoses are not spun out of thin air. You acquire a sense of what is so, and what will be declared later to be proven and agreed to be so. This knowing is not so much psychic as it is integrative; it involves piecing together a lot of different kinds of information into a pattern that makes sense. Imagine having a jigsaw puzzle that only has 25 percent of the puzzle pieces. As you begin to lay the pieces out, a picture starts to appear. At some point, even though you don't have all the pieces, the image will become recognizable with the right pair of eyes. The conclusion reached is based on a scattering of bits of data, and cannot be in any way considered a proven conclusion in either legal or scientific terms. It may become proven later, when more of the puzzle is laid out; but now it is in the "pre-knowing" stage. Much of integrative and holistic medicine occupies this area of pre-knowing.

I have been either blessed (or cursed) with this kind of pre-knowing for much of my life: blessed because it has been very exciting to find my way into areas of science before they become popular or even accepted; cursed, because I have done studies and tried to get funding in several areas many years before the ideas became acceptable or before the techniques to do good studies had been developed. For instance, I left one area of interest, "psycho-immunology," eight years before it was renamed psycho-neuro-immunology and became an acceptable field of study.

All of us have this skill to some degree, and its accuracy depends on how many different types of data we personally integrate. For example, I knew that cigarettes caused cancer and disease nearly 50 years ago, and so did most people. Teens back then called cigarettes "cancer sticks," and smoked them anyway. Doctors smoked while they saw patients. Non-smokers were constantly subjected to incredible levels of secondary smoke in buses, homes, restaurants, and offices. My own mother chained smoked for 50 years. But there was no official proof of this association for decades to come, and the cigarette companies told dying smokers there was no proof cigarettes contributed to their emphysema and lung cancer despite an article in the British Medical Journal in 1950 showing this association. Science could not yet prove the link, and the courts would not support it until the Tobacco Master Settlement Agreement in 1998. How did the general population know for decades what the medical authorities and the legal system officially did not?

In medical school, the pathologist at Bellevue would present us with a pair of black lungs with fish-meat-like lumps. He would ask us to guess the patient's history, and we would say, "WWII veteran, fifty-year-old chronic smoker with lung cancer." "Right!" he would say. But what clinched the knowing at that time was that overwhelming circumstantial evidence, epidemiologic data, animal and test tube scientific studies, folk knowledge, and case histories all pointed toward the relationship. So I had a lot of folk, clinical, and basic science data leading to my "knowing" that smoking caused lung disease. And although there was no absolute proof in a scientific or legal sense, so too, did a lot of the population at large.

Why am I hammering on smoking in a book on skin? Aside from the fact that smoking ages the skin, what I am really getting at is that there are dozens of other habits and environmental exposures today that are just as insidious and harmful as smoking. Directly or indirectly, many of these habits harm the skin and the body. From an official scientific and legal standpoint, the risks of these habits are unknown or overlooked. They all have two critical aspects in common. First, we are in one way or another addicted to the process or products involved, both as individuals and as a society. Second, there are large financial benefits involved in providing those processes or products. Both of these factors make the individual and collective brain go foggy. Our thinking gets soft and mushy, and we wind up doing lots of dangerous, foolish things to ourselves and our environment for decades before we get smart. Doctors who speak out about these things are often labeled "quacks" and challenged by medical boards and insurance companies while millions of people continue to suffer.

What other things did my colleagues in alternative medicine know before they became official? In 1983, our small seminal holistic group had a legendary meeting on essential fatty acids. Many of the 30 or 40 attendees and presenters later became well known in either popular or holistic circles. Robert Atkins (of

The Atkins Diet fame) attended and David Horrobin (one of the premier researchers into the anti-inflammatory effects of evening primrose oil and gamma-linolenic acid) and Jeff Bland (the father of functional medicine) presented. Anti- and pro-inflammatory essential fatty acids and their metabolic pathways and the damaging effects of partially hydrogenated oils were clearly described and documented. The public has been duped into believing they were improving their health by switching to margarine and other partially hydrogenated oil-containing products as a staple in their diets. Unfortunately, it took nearly 24 years before the voices of alternative medicine practitioners were heard and the common industrial process of putting partially hydrogenated (trans-saturated) oils into foods finally became a matter of public understanding and outcry. Because of this lag, a whole extra generation of humans got the harmful effects of accumulating these adulterated oils in their body tissues!

It is true that these synthetic fats play an important role in extending shelf life and preventing the fats in baked goods from becoming rancid. Less food is thrown away, and rancid oil is worse than partially hydrogenated. We love being able to eat that piece of cake which has been in the cupboard for a week. The food industry loves the nine-month shelf life for baked and other goods, without refrigeration. The Society of Oil Chemists was not evil when it came out in favor of these oils. But incorporating these partially hydrogenated fats as a significant part of our diets has rendered them a significant component of our cell membranes and body tissues, and it's taking a toll on the function of our skin, arteries, and brain.

I have moved in the direction of natural and holistic medicine because it moves away from those artificial "body ecology disasters" by understanding what exposures can be harmful. I place my trust in wisdom handed down over centuries and in substances that mammals have been eating for millions of years. Avoidance of environmental toxins, allergens, and other aggravators is essential for restoring normal body function.

My own scientific studies at the NIH led me to understand the role of cross-reactivity in lymphocyte immunity, and the implications it has on the factors which could incite inflammation in the body. This will be explained in greater detail later (see Chapter 4). Here my point is the tremendous health cost and financial cost resulting from the length of the time that passes between initial scientific understanding of a concept and application to improving health. It took 22 years from the publication of our first NIH paper in 1977 to the publication of the article in the *New England Journal of Medicine* in December of 1999 on cross-reactivity and molecular mimicry and its role in disease (molecular mimicry occurs when a particular chemical, bacteria or virus closely resembles another part of an individual's biochemical makeup). Many physicians today still do not incorporate the clinical implications of these findings into their practice. In other words, it took almost a generation before the concept we gleaned from our experiments were further generalized and published in a top clinical journal where more erudite physicians could have access to it. Even now, this important concept is not part of the majority thinking among doctors.

For me, alternative medicine involves discovering and helping individuals find out what molecular mimics are getting their immune systems so riled up that they attack their own tissues with inflammation. I look at causes and treatment as a doctor, and then I look again as an alternative physician with a kind of pre-knowing that attempts to peer through the collective mind fog with a more sensible view on what the human body can tolerate. I understand that learned authorities in powerful positions are extremely wary of my thinking because of the lack of adequate randomized control studies. To them, I am the one with fuzzy thinking. But maybe, just as video cameras that can create a clear picture from a shaky camera (known as fuzzy logic), I am the one with the fuzzy logic that produces a focused picture from shaky data.

Another example of this has to do with mercury fillings in our teeth. Dentists were only doing what they had learned as the standard of practice in dentistry, when they filled cavities using a silver-mercury amalgam. They were helping people by fixing their teeth with fillings that lasted for decades. However, in more recent years alternative practitioners, including me, and the health systems in various other countries, have been concerned about the harmful effects of mercury to our bodies and to our environment. When mercury enters the air from coal-fired power plants and is in the water from mining operations, it accumulates in fish to levels that make fish unsuitable for consumption more frequently than once a month by pregnant women and small children. While mercury fillings are still legal in the United States, they've been banned in Norway, Sweden, and Denmark. In the United States, dentists can't throw mercury down the sink because it is considered a hazardous waste, but they are allowed to put it inside your teeth. Mercury can poison various organs in the body including the brain and digestive system. What makes it OK to be used inside your mouth? This is just one of the many health fiascos imbedded in our culture, health, political and economic environment. As in numerous other issues, our societal system is too unwieldy to tackle this paradox for the health of our people.

What Will We Wish We Had "Known" Twenty Years from Now?

Conventional dermatologists today do some great detective work, looking for what is causing disease. Occupational medicine and its relationship to contact dermatitis and the search for infectious, molecular, and genetic causes of disease are just a few examples of excellence in clinical and research dermatology we should all seek. But they often dismiss dietary contributions to disease. They don't often look at the role of the digestive system and the liver, or the role of toxicity from the 80,000 chemicals in common use today. They tend to ignore the role of heavy metals, the overgrowth of organisms in the digestive tract, and the influence of environmental exposures. All these things are possible causative factors of skin disease today. These factors that destroy our systems, and cause break-outs in our skin in the process, are the challenges left to be dealt with by the holistic dermatologist. That is what I want to tell you about in this book, so that you can more clearly see your options for clearing your skin condition when your dermatologist sees only how to calm the process down and not how to find and resolve the cause.

Most important is that many of the causes of skin conditions are known or can be deduced from a broad pattern of information that is known today. The answers may be individual-specific, may not have adequate proof, and may be controversial as far as the medical literature is concerned; but piecing together a careful history, combing the scientific data in cells and humans, as well as the lore **of different healing traditions** often yields helpful insights into how to reverse a specific skin problem. This is the best way a doctor who is versed in medicine, medical science, and alternative approaches, can then identify the underlying causes and reverse the skin conditions.

CHAPTER 3

DEMONS OF THE MIND: THE ROOTS OF ILLNESS

Anthony's Warts

Anthony was a young lawyer, in clerkship at a local law firm, who worked hard and was religious. But he had a minor skin problem that would not go away with conventional treatment, and he was paralyzed in his healing by a dark secret which bothered him every time he was confronted with his rash. He had two types of genital warts, which although small, just would not respond to freezing or scraping. His pain was that these had appeared after doing something in a weak moment that was completely out of character for him: he had had sex with a prostitute. From a moral, religious, and hygienic point of view as a lawyer, this was all wrong for him, and the warts reminded him that although he had done this only once, it was something for which he could never forgive himself.

I worked with him to strengthen his immunity to fight off the warts, and I repeatedly scraped off the warts surgically. But more important, I worked with Anthony to get him to forgive himself for his past action, so that he could summon his healing energy to reject the warts and move on from this place of being stuck. At the psychological and emotional level, he could see how his guilt and shame could contribute to the persistence of his warts, but he could not stop feeling these emotions for what he had done. His best option was to pray for a release from these feelings, for an ability to forgive himself, so that he could heal and move on. Anthony was earnest in his prayer, and began to release his shame and self-criticism. His lesions began to diminish with removal, coming back more and more slowly until, after some months, he was feeling better about himself and was clear of recurrent genital warts. He had freed himself of a skin condition that had stood as a mark of his shame. And he was now able to consider resuming a normal social life for a young single male.

Healing here was a combination of conventional surgical treatment, herbal support, and transformational release directed at mental and emotional issues with a spiritual approach. I believe that the spiritual release was crucial for allowing Anthony's system to stop punishing him, and instead allow his immune system to fight off his viral warts. He certainly was not getting any better when he was being treated only by wart removal.

The Weaving

There is a lot of information in the medical literature on the relationship between mental, emotional, and spiritual issues and disease. More specifically, there was a conference on stress and the skin a few years ago in which data was presented to show relationships between stress and skin disease at every level measurable. This went from population studies, to illustration of nerve effects on immune cells in the skin, to molecular messages, to the immune system related to brain activity. There are many different emotional and psychological difficulties that can influence the immune system and they can do so by a variety of mechanisms. In some instances, emotional conflicts can directly or indirectly influence the immune system and subsequently cause skin disease. From a holistic viewpoint, it's useful to search for psychological and emotional conditions that can lead to illness when a condition does not respond to ordinary treatment.

Extraordinary healing best happens when all the contributing factors are corrected together. I have found that I connect with some people in such a way as to be able to bring them along this path in a wonderful way. Sometimes it involves guiding them to therapists or onto a spiritual path they are already familiar with; I provide a gentle push to do the work they know deep down they must do.

This work can be highly personal, and people only reach a point where their emotional issues manifest physical illness in conjunction with a lot of environmental and genetic factors over a period of many years. So I am not able to make this connection with everyone who comes to me, and I can only pray that those who need transformation at those non-physical levels find someone else who can guide them on their path, or find the inner wisdom to do it on their own.

I have had many experiences that have convinced me that mental, emotional, and spiritual problems contribute to illness, and that for some people, addressing them is an important component for healing.

Plagued with anxiety, allergies, and earaches as a child, I grew up with a sense that somehow my emotional discomfort was related to being sick so much. My parents had a book on psychosomatic illness that I read as a young boy, confirming my feelings. In my training I came across two compendiums from a series of conferences at the NY Academy of Science on Psychosomatic Factors in Cancer, published in 1968 and 1969. These became a kind of "bible" for me in learning about emotional effect on immunity and disease. I went on to meet some of the key authors, wrote a grant for studying the effects of emotional shock on immune function, and eventually conducted research studies on the effect of emotional factors on immunity in cancer and in contact dermatitis.

Another Example: Helena's Zoster

A young woman named Helena came to me for a painful rash on the face. She had been under enormous pressure since her mother died in a foreign country, and was aggravated by the messy aftermath of a contested will. Indeed, she was still quietly tumbling with the torment of both the loss and the ensuing acrimony and financial loss. But she was tough, and all that showed from this harrowing experience was the rash on her face.

Helena's rash was just on one side, and with the pain and the blisters it was not hard to diagnose her as having shingles, caused by the herpes zoster virus. She only wanted natural treatment, and my combination of amino acids and vitamins worked very nicely in zoster. But something about her rash had me very concerned. You see, there was a small blister on the tip of her nose. That indicates involvement of the ophthalmic branch of the fifth cranial nerve, which means that it is likely to involve the cornea of the eye as well. The destructive process caused by herpes zoster and the damaging vasculitis which occurs after, causes eye problems and may cause blindness. I suggested that in this case, she consider one of the antiviral medications that are known to stop the virus and prevent further spread of the virus to the eye.

She refused any pharmaceuticals, and refused to see an eye specialist, despite my repeated warnings about the danger involved. So I added an energetic technique, NeuroModulation Technique (NMT), to my treatment plan. This is a method for resetting autonomic function using instructive affirmation along with tapping down the acupuncture meridians along the spine, in different phases of breathing. In the process, I instructed her immune system to clear the virus. I also found, as expected, that she had mental patterns interfering with the ability of her immune system to control the virus. I tapped down her spine with an instruction to clear these "pernicious synaptic patterns" related to her emotional trauma which were interfering with her recovery.

She left, happy with all my treatment. I tried to call her a week later, because I was very concerned about her eye. I could not reach her to get a phone follow-up, as she had left the country. But I got a call later, telling me that her rash had cleared nicely after the last appointment, and that she was doing well.

The Roots of Illness

When a disease-producing habit, such as stuffing emotional pain with sweets, comes up again and again in preventing healing of a condition, it is time to explore and attempt to heal the psychological and emotional aspects of that individual. When circumstances reveal that it is impossible to find such a healing within the "realities" of that individual's situation, it is time to seek an answer on the spiritual plane. So many of the ills of both individuals and our life on this planet have that level of impossibility; in such cases we can only begin to approach a holistic solution by seeking answers at the spiritual level.

There are many dysfunctional ways of coping with past trauma that people discover on their own, at some low point in their lives, while struggling with habits or compulsions that lead to disease. There is a spiritual emptiness that comes when blotting out unacceptable inner pain by destructive habit. The other side of this dysfunctional pattern is the opportunity to discover the specific unconscious pain that is emerging, and furthermore, to develop a spiritual life in the process of over-coming it.

Whether it is entering a 12-step program such as AA for drinking issues, or praying in the quiet of one's own sacred space or place of worship, there is a time, when a skin problem has underlying issues which cannot be solved, to ask for a new level of answers one was not previously ready to hear.

Where do we find these answers?

There are guidelines for our ways in the loving words of the Sages of the great Religions and Schools of Wisdom. Because these benevolent teachings encom-pass the heart and soul of health on this planet and our joyful emanation into the Universe, they can guide our choices for the sustained well-being of the individual and of life on this planet. More and more, the imperative for a renewable future requires us to re-think the choices we make as individuals and as a society, if our present is to be sweet, and our future is to become present. The accelerated pace of unsustainable choices—selling off our future for a juicier treat in the moment—is catching up with us as rapidly as a lit fuse. Lip service and watered-down efforts will not keep the flames of our short-sighted hypocrisy from reaching our doorstep. For example, we must each wrestle with the desires for immediate gratification versus long-term health. At a societal level, we must wrestle with the conflict between the fiduciary responsibilities of corporations to show profit yearly versus the spiritual dictum of the sins of the father reaching down unto the 7th generation. Never before in the history of our species could the errors of poor planning on a global level accelerate chronic disease or lead quickly to impossible environmental burdens and loss of options for continued human life on Earth as is the case now. Only a truly soul-searching plea to the Loving Spirit that resides within the heart of every man will enable us to make the right choice at every fork in the road, as individuals and as a species.

Working back along the chain of causes to the origin of illness, one inevitably comes to disturbances in the mind, emotions, or spirit. This is not to say that infections, genetic conditions, susceptibilities, and injuries beyond one's control don't lead to skin disease. But many of a person's choices are made simply to quiet inner pain and conflict. From stuffing oneself with the wrong foods, or too much food, to push down an emotion or thought, to taking chances at a pick-up bar, skin conditions may reflect inner emotions and thoughts which steer a person away from the best choice for the whole being. There are many stories of people whose skin diseases have healed through mind-directed therapy. Contributing factors from the emotions are not always quite clear to the skin disease sufferer. For example, the severe itching and scratching cycle that some skin disease patients suffer could also be an excellent distraction from even more uncomfortable emotional conflicts they are avoiding.

Methods of Treatment:

Sometimes, the first step to clearing hidden issues impacting one's health is to identify what those issues are. Keeping a journal, writing down one's thoughts, reactions, and dreams, is a good start. Engaging in a meditation practice in which you quiet your mind and sit, dismissing other thoughts, gives you an opportunity to see what bubbles up from the unconscious mind.

- **Meditation**: Meditation, while a simple process, is by no means easy. Don't let this intimidate you; anyone can learn to meditate by practicing a technique that works for them. Many people learn in a group, from a teacher, who instructs students in a particular technique and can guide you through the challenges that come from trying to tame the mind. Some people use audio recordings to guide them on meditative journeys. While it is theoretically possible to learn from a book and recording, most people find that in-person guidance leads to more effective meditation. It may be most beneficial to learn a technique from a teacher, and then practice on one's own, with periodic meetings with your teacher or teachers, with guidance from books and fellow meditators, to supplement the practice.

The essence of meditation is understanding that you, as a being, are more than the thoughts in your mind. You will learn that your mind has well-worn habits (for example, the habit for some is worry) that may detract from healing or being who you really are. Meditation is a tool for observing the mind and quieting the reactions to one's thoughts, using a as the breath, the sensations, or a word or phrase. In the well-developed traditions of meditation from India, this word or phrase is called a "mantra," and specific mantras are either taught for their meaning, or chosen by a teacher for a student to use. To meditate, sit upright and keep bringing your focus of attention back to the word you have chosen, or to the sensation of your breath moving through your nostrils. Meditation can work to root out suffering by clearing one's attachment to living in the past or future, to avoiding pain and craving pleasure. When one experiences the present moment without attachment, one is relieved from the cycle of suffering and thus connected to the deeper, unchanging realm of peacefulness.

The agitated mind has a tendency to wander from thought to thought, similarly to a curious monkey swinging from vine to vine. Meditation is the process of bringing your mind back gently to the original focus, again and again, each time it wanders. Gentleness is most important, so that you do not criticize yourself for having difficulty with staying focused, which is simply another way of letting the mind wander. Increased skill comes with practice. With that comes an awareness of where your mind is wandering, as well as an increased ability to keep focused. Even more important, even if for only fleeting moments at first, is a great feeling of inner calm that is the experience of the real you. It is out of that calm that you begin to experience who you are. Your entire system calms down. Organs that are racing to the tune of an anxious mind begin to slow down and get a much-needed rest. As your mind becomes steadier, your outward appearance expresses this steadiness. Choices can be made which truly support the health of the skin and body.

The mantras from various spiritual and religious traditions or teachers have a further role, if you choose to use them. They have the ability to expand your sense of who you are and what you are capable of. If you have a rash, with scratching fits, and it is being caused by a painful internal conflict, it is crucial to expand your perspective. Expanding your concept of who you are and what your inborn capabilities are is like opening a deeper level of the software that was already installed in your computer. A mantra or affirmation can remind you that you are a unique manifestation of the Universe and make possible for you a new level of understanding the larger you. A series of such thoughts opens you to a much wider concept of the miracles in your life and the miraculous possibilities that can exist for you. Many authors have drawn from ancient religious and spiritual teachings and their own experience in that light, and developed guidance for this path of meditation.

If your meditation leads to recurrent thoughts that are disturbing, or might lead to harm to yourself or others, it is important to seek professional help via a psychologist, psychiatrist, or other qualified helper. Look at this as a clear identification of a problem and a path to a level of treatment that can bring about resolution. We all carry different levels of neurochemical stresses, mental trauma, and poor habits in dealing with them. When all those come together in the wrong way, the results can be destructive. You need to identify this and find help getting through it.

Some meditation techniques that you can explore include Vipassana, or Insight Meditation, Transcendental Meditation, Zen Buddhist meditation, mindfulness, etc. Exploring a variety of forms of meditation will help you discover the one that works best for you. Once you have found your style, do your best to make it a daily practice and not to mix different forms of meditation. Guidance from teachers can strengthen your practice. This helps you go deeper and deeper within your practice and get the most benefit.

Taking time to get free of the stories from our mind can be a great way to heal old patterns which have been holding you down in your illness.

- **Therapy:** Psychologists and therapists can often be of help with conflicts and issues that are hard to resolve. There are new schools of therapy that can be very effective in helping you work through blind spots when you are too close to your problem to see it clearly. These include, for example, placing an imaginary difficult person from your past in a chair and telling them what you have always wanted, but have been unable, to say. Or picturing a particularly painful episode in your earlier life, and changing the story in a way that empowers you.

  Finding the right therapist is a very individual process. It's important to identify what you want to get from therapy, and then develop criteria for choosing the person who will help you best achieve your goal. Some questions you might ask yourself when interviewing different therapists are: "Could I trust this person?" "Could I tell this person difficult things about myself and not be judged?" "Does this person have valuable insight and wisdom?" "Will this person be honest with me and challenge me in a healthy way so that I can grow?" "Will this person help me to make my own life decisions and distinctions?"

  Some modes of therapy include Gestalt therapy, behavioral psychology, integrative therapy, drama therapy, co-counseling, and grief counseling.

• **Support Groups and 12-Step Recovery Groups:** There are also all sorts of support groups for people with various issues. These issues can range from situational issues such as having a relative with Alzheimer' Disease, to coming from a dysfunctional family, or having an addiction to food or alcohol. When destructive acting-out behaviors are occurring, it is difficult to address the underlying issues until you put some distance between you and the behaviors.

When you can lay out the dilemma in your life and there is clearly no solution to the problem any rational person can provide for you, it is time to seek help from a higher level. Twelve-step groups direct you to seek help from a Higher Power of your choice, and do not require any specific religious belief. The 12-step groups are one model of a group that works for people, but by no means are the only one. It is worth attending meetings more than once and exploring more than one group to find whether you have arrived in the right place. These meetings offer a method of managing one's difficulties without resorting to old behavior, of finding what parts of your underlying personality and history contribute to the problem, and of letting go. They also offer the support of others with whom you can share your struggle more comfortably than even with friends or relatives who do not share the same struggles. Twelve-step groups are always free (usually people donate a couple of dollars when they attend a meeting) and so offer an incredible amount of resources for almost no money, for as long as you find them beneficial. As you correct destructive behaviors, the mind and the body often correct themselves very easily.

Some kinds of twelve-step groups include Alcoholics Anonymous, Al-anon, Co-dependents Anonymous, Overeaters Anonymous, Marijuana Anonymous, Debtors Anonymous, Sex Addicts Anonymous, and even a group called Clutterers Anonymous, for those who collect too many possessions.

Physical and Emotional Healing

Talking about one's issues can be incredibly beneficial, but sometimes talk is just that. When we've got everything well-analyzed, but nothing in our lives is changing, physical healing may be required. Often, in combination with therapy or a support group, some kind of physical healing can help a person move through seemingly immovable problems.

When we are young, we develop a system of beliefs that help us make sense of and survive our world. Often, they help us cope with dysfunction in our families or in society. As we become adults, we may find that the very systems that helped us survive begin to cause us pain and suffering. These beliefs are held in the background of our unconscious mind, and don't manifest themselves as beliefs we can just change by changing our minds. We've already tried that. They manifest themselves as a way of being in life, and through what our lives look and feel like. Letting go of old beliefs that no longer serve us through non-verbal healing can be a refreshing change of pace for many people.

Some methods of physical and emotional healing techniques include massage, acupuncture, craniosacral therapy, yoga, qi gong, chiropractic, and Feldenkrais therapy. Particular movements of the physical body can bring up and release locked-in trauma for some people. More expensive is not necessarily better. Getting a referral from a friend who is a satisfied customer is a great way to find a quality practitioner. Try more than one until you find who's right for you.

You'll find that each form of healthy behavior enhances the body's ability to improve itself. For example, taking up yoga a few times a week could improve your mental health such that it may eventually have a positive effect on your chronic skin condition.

Spiritual Healing: Medical Intuitives, Psychic Healers, Prayer Healers, and Shamans

There are many other forms of spiritual healing and healers out there. Exploring spiritual healing can be a strange new world full of possibility and wonder, extraordinary claims, and sometimes extraordinary miracles. I will discuss a few examples of this healing, and give you some important guidelines that I believe will keep you out of trouble in your search.

Be Wary of the Cult

First of all, the cost of such healing should be up front and apparent soon, if not initially. There is no such thing as completely free help. I would be concerned with any path that demands no money but costs you your "soul" when committing to a leader, group, guru, or path. You may want to get better, but that seems a heavy price to pay to free your burden. So be sure that you know what you are getting into and that you are really willing to pay the price. Note that many spiritual paths do require real commitment and firm guidance to achieve the full benefit; but you should always retain personal choice and authority about what you think and feel, and what is right for you and when.

Healer Bruno Groening

Bruno Groening was a healer in Germany in the 1940s and 1950s, who would come into a town and heal, for example, a sick child who did not respond to medical therapy. Soon, others came to be healed, and at times he would have ten thousand people in the town square for a healing. People who were healed by him purportedly took on the ability to heal others. As you might expect, the medical authorities banned him from doing his healings and he died in exile in Paris.

However, his methods lived on. One of the people who had been healed, and had the ability to heal others, began forming a group of her own. Soon more and more groups were formed, each carefully documenting the healings that had occurred. Today there are more than a thousand groups throughout the world using his methods. An earnest group with a good leader can be very helpful, and can even spark dramatic changes in the health of some participants. The Groening group is supported by donations and sales of literature. The only mandate is to collect accurate reports of healings and have a physician document and review the results for publication in their journal. I think the commitment cost is quite reasonable; but clearly, if you are healed, you may want to help with the organization, healing others, and this is a commitment to consider.

Healing Forces

Anyone who either believes in God or is willing to try to do so, can be a healer using Bruno's method. The basic method is very straightforward (if you are an atheist reading this, I suggest you just ponder and address the magnificence of the Universe). First, sit in a relaxed, upright position. Uncross your hands and feet, and place your hands, palms upward, on your knees. I like to use a progressive relaxation exercise to begin, gradually bringing my attention from my toes upward, through each part of my body, until I reach my face. You can focus on your breathing, inspirational music, or anything that will bring you into a relaxed and meditative state of mind. Then ask God to send the "healing force" through you. Keep that request in your mind, and become aware of your sensations. You may experience a sensation resembling a tingling running up your leg and through your body, or some other sensation. Once in that state of request, you can ask for healing of yourself, your family, your friends, community, country, or planet or anyone else you wish. You can go through your list of who you are asking to be healed each time, including yourself. You do not have to tell God how you want that healing to be done; the Divine Intelligence of the Universe can handle that problem. Some people who get healed have a temporary aggravation of symptoms, which have been termed "regulations." These are not unlike the "healing crises" seen in some forms of herbal treatment, or the aggravations of symptoms seen with homeopathic treatment. Such aggravations should last only a few days and then give way to improvement of your condition. If not, you should seek medical help to see what else is going on, and seek help from a Bruno therapy group to make sure you are on the right path.

A number of really miraculous cures have been documented by physicians who have examined patients and their records carefully and then had other physicians review them for accuracy. Contemplating the reality of such healings is a powerful stimulus for opening up to the possibility of your own miraculous cure. It does not happen for everyone, but it clearly happens for some. Some people visualize Bruno Groening, or even ask his help to bring healing. I have been reassured by key people in the program that although such visualization may help, it is by no means a requirement for the healing.

Many different religions and spiritual paths have a history of saints, healers, healing prayers, and connections with the Divine to bring about healing. You may already see similarity between Bruno's healing and another method. If there is another method which is closer to your own Spiritual or Religious beliefs, I encourage you to fly upward on its inspiration and use it to help with your healing and becoming who you want to be.

Other Healers

There are a number of people who claim to have been helped or healed by people in this category. I have met various healers who seem like honest people, who claim to do this work. I think that this kind of help should be approached carefully, with good recommendation by people you trust who have had personal experience with the healer. I think that this work should also supplement care directed at the physical realm of your problem. If a healer tells you to stop your other forms of care, that would be a red flag to me about the degree to which they are control freaks, and about their credibility in general.

A friend of mine had a bad knee fixed by a South American Shaman, whose payment plan consisted of putting a donation into his tin can. When she went back to Brazil the next year to fix her other knee, she went to someone who demanded payment right away. She paid and was treated but the second treatment was of no help for her knee. The money-focused shaman was apparently not the real thing, and his focus, in that culture at that time, should have revealed his intentions.

Sometimes, the healing ability comes to a person of deep belief and practice only at certain times when they get in touch with that belief. My wife gave a workshop on spiritual healing at a religious conference a few years ago. We were early arriving at our assigned room, which was a lovely large room set up as a Zen meditation classroom. Being her assistant in such a situation, I insisted that we set up the lapel microphone and sound system for her so that people in the room could hear. We were early and there wasn't a soul around waiting for the class, and she thought it would be unnecessary for the few people who might show up to hear her. I emphasize this, as her "assistant" in this situation, to provide a sense of her incredible modesty regarding her gifts.

Eventually, the classroom began to fill up and she began her instructions. First, she explained that all healing came from the Universal Force, and it was God that you asked to do the healing. When doing healing, she explained, you make yourself a channel for God's healing to come through. Then she instructed people on how to lay on hands to heal. The key part was to put the intention to heal throughout your being, and extend this into your hands, with feeling that the healing would emerge from them (DO try this at home). The first volunteer had a chronic pain in his neck. She placed her hands on his neck with intention to heal, and he said the pain went away. I held the mike up to his mouth and asked him to repeat that for the rest of the group there. She then asked the class to pair up, identify an area of the body that needed healing, and send healing energy from one to another in each pair. I found myself joining in the spiritual fun, and healing people with whom I was paired, almost as naturally as riding a bicycle.

Later that evening, some word of my ability to heal had apparently gotten around, and I was approached by a woman who asked me to treat her. She was scheduled to sing a key segment in the evening program, and she had lost her voice during practice. Apparently, the piano player was playing too loudly, and she didn't have a mike; she sang louder than her vocal cords could sustain. She had laryngitis, with a program to perform in three hours. I was both honored and humbled, and without much thought, I brought my intention to healing and my focus on the energy in my hands. I placed them near her throat, and sent what I pictured to be healing energy, as I had done in the class a few hours earlier. I had no expectations; I simply did what I had done before. I went to the musical program that evening and heard her sing a beautiful jazz set with the piano player for 45 minutes. Either she had a spontaneous cure, or the healing energy that I carried from the class had something to do with her voice returning. Honestly, I don't myself believe that I alone brought about the healing. It is easier for me to believe that I was a kind of "channel" for healing from Source, guided by my wife's access to that Source, in that class of seekers and believers who came for a weekend of spiritual growth.

I am saying this not just to minimize my own healing abilities, but more to emphasize that situation, context, and presence of people who are believers and seekers; earnest guides are all-important for spiritual healing to occur. I am also mentioning this to say that in the right circumstances, many of those who are reading this now can do healing, just as I did. I set the intention to heal, being taught by a successful healer and having a certain casual confidence. The person to be healed was both receptive, and confident in my healing ability, having heard that I had healed others she knew. Many healers keep themselves in that healing state on a regular basis, which makes their work more effective. But there is a special equation that involves both the healer and the person to be healed, their surrounding circumstances, and the particular time that the healing is attempted.

How Does Emotional "Healing" Work?

We come into this world with not only the genetic material of our parents, but some sort of energetic imprint of their state of being and of the experiences our mother has during our journey in her womb. If she is happy and well nourished, we get different information for the construction of our nervous and immune systems than if she is poorly nourished, repeatedly traumatized, or living in fear or depression. This same kind of signaling goes on during our infancy and childhood, conditioning how we feel inside. By the time we grow up, we may have numerous areas of internal conflict and pain of which we are barely conscious. They rule us, in that we take all sorts of measures to avoid experiencing them. These feelings may be completely submerged below our awareness. Or they may be like icebergs, barely showing on the surface but seething away underneath. They are often given away by overreactions to small or annoying incidents, or we may experience emotional twinges, with the majority of the issue floating beneath the surface of our awareness.

Often, we have developed patterns, habits, obsessions, or addictions to take us away from the pain of experiencing these emotions or anything that brings them up. These patterns may be initially pleasurable, but ultimately self-destructive. Eating a container of ice cream or drinking a bottle of wine can take away the pain that conflicted situations or painful memories bring. So can scratching of an itch to the point of bleeding. Psychological, emotional, and spiritual techniques, when they touch and release the core of the problem, not only break the habit cycle contributing to the domino sequence of the disease, they also free up a tremendous amount of energy from inappropriate informational signaling at every level of your body. Molecular, cellular, organ, and overall central nervous system-directed information influences how all the complex network of you functions. Releasing inner trauma, forgiving yourself, or coming into appreciation of the good things in your life can be like breaking through a cocoon in which you were trapped, allowing the butterfly of your soul to take flight on a path your former self could never dream of. This is stuff of miraculous cures. And it is possible and available to you and to those who seek it. Transformation and release on the inside while making changes to counter underlying physical factors is a very potent prescription. Combined with the right therapeutic supplements, medical care or other methods, results can be obtained where none are thought to exist. This does not happen for everyone, but it is a path to resolution for some who are told that there is none. And there are many benefits from just walking that path.

If your rational mind is now resisting the assertion that emotional release could change your body's physiology, its chemical operation, let me shed some light on what is known. For years I was interested in the effects of stress on immune function, and found studies showing such a link in disorders as far apart as acne, eczema, psoriasis, cancer, arthritis, and bowel disease. However, I later found out by personal experience how difficult it was to conduct truly scientific studies in this area.

After my internship, I made a point of visiting some of the major researchers in psychosomatic illness in the country. The first was Dr. George Engel, at the medical school of my former alma mater, the University of Rochester. He led a group which had been started by Dr. John Romano, which focused on many different aspects of the influence of the mind on the body and disease. One of the most graphic illustrations of psychosomatic effects was a patient with a fistula (tube) opening that allowed doctors to look directly into the patient's stomach. They could see differences in color as blood was brought to the stomach during emotional experiences. Less than a decade after my visit, Dr. Robert Ader at that center was able to demonstrate conditioning of an immune response in mice. This brought the study of psychological effects on immune function to a new level of scientific validity. When I met Dr. George Solomon in California, I was able to help interpret some of the studies he had done in which mice carrying out their aggression were healthier than those that did not, based on the concept that aggressive activity released growth hormone that then improved immune responses. It was also where I felt validated using the term, "psycho-immunology," as Dr. Solomon was using the same term to describe the relationship between the mind and the immune system.

This still left open the question about how these psychological factors could change immune and other physiologic responses. I was fortunate to hear and meet another scientist who uncovered perhaps the greatest understanding of this link. Candice Pert was a very accomplished neuroscientist at the NIH, with nearly 200 scientific articles to her credit. She had been identifying molecules related to various emotional states. A very important emotion came over her when she met and later married an immunologist. Together, they gave the connection between emotions and immune function a whole new level of validity, and made the field of psycho-neuro-immunology scientifically plausible (this story is much better told in her book, *The Molecules of Emotion*). Simply stated, different emotional states cause release of chemical signals that influence changes in the immune system and other systems to either favor or suppress disease. Finally, with her study results, my belief that one's mind and thoughts influence immunity and skin disease was proven to a greater degree scientifically.

Summary

Working on your physical system and mental-emotional-spiritual realm are mutually beneficial activities. If any "spiritual healer" tries to tell you otherwise, they probably do not belong on your healing team.

There are wonderful opportunities to heal your skin condition even if diet change and other natural treatments are not sufficient. Your skin disorder can be a symptom and visible sign to let others know that something deep inside you needs to heal so that you can live your life to the fullest. If you consume unhealthy foods to "stuff a hole in your soul," perhaps you will find a healthier way to fill that hole. If your thoughts are on work worries while you eat rather than on your food, you have an opportunity to change this, not only to improve your digestion and inflammation, but also to bring a new level of enjoyment and equanimity to your life. If your depression is what slows the function of your immune system, you have a chance to change this and therefore feel better and live a more healthy life. The opportunity to live out the most exciting level of your soul's journey is within you and sometimes just a prayer away. Certainly there are many paths and treatments that can restore you to a more peaceful relationship with yourself. You deserve to overcome the obstacles and make your life more vibrant. Consider that the emotionally triggered skin condition may serve as a bookmark in your life to remind you how much richer your life can be if you clear your inner turmoil. Find the guides and programs you need and you may be surprised by the overall improvement in your skin and your well-being.

CHAPTER 4
YOUR SKIN ON FIRE: INFLAMMATION AND THE SKIN

Inflammation and the Body's Defense System, Illustrated

Imagine waking up on a camping trip feeling your leg on fire. The day before, you hiked through the woods, got cut up on branches and briars, and feel asleep from exhaustion when you got back to camp. When you look at your leg in the daylight, you see scratches and a bright red, hot, swollen, tender rash. Your skin is "on fire," or "in flame." We use the term "*in flame*-ation" or inflammation to describe such a condition. But what could have caused it, and what can you do about it? Finding out what kind of rash it is and what caused it will help you determine how best to reduce the inflammation. The wrong guess could mean a delay to proper treatment. If the cause is an infection, that delay could put your leg and you at risk. If it is from an allergy, different treatment and other concerns are factors.

In many cases, success in treating skin disease is only obtained after making changes to bring multiple body systems into balance and restore a more normal function. We are constantly learning about more components of our immune systems that play a role in an immune response against self that can potentially be modified to treat skin inflammation. Successes in my practice tell me that treating lifestyle and diet issues can modify immune factors to allow motivated people to put out the fire of inflammation in their skin and avoid other more dangerous and invasive forms of therapy.

One of most exciting realizations for me is that understanding the path of activation of different branches of the immune system gives us a way to identify and remove triggers that are setting off an immune reaction leading to an inflammatory skin disease. Removing triggers has the possibility of stopping the skin condition without having to use immunosuppressants, avoiding the "collateral damage" that often results from use of such powerful and broad-reaching weapons from our pharmacologic arsenal. Understanding the immune system in a functional way enables us to prescribe lifestyle and nutritional changes that relate to patients' day-to-day experiences.

Many skin conditions have inflammation as part of their cause, where the immune system is attacking in the area of the rash, even though they are not so obviously red, hot, or swollen. The kind and location of the inflammatory attack, and the location in the skin at which it is occurring, determines the kind of skin condition that we see. Understanding this helps us to better understand how to control skin disorders, what kind of testing to do, and how to look deeper for answers to challenging problems. Also helpful is exploring in depth the immunology literature when re-evaluating what dermatologists learn, teach, and generally regard as the actual cause of specific skin conditions. The frequency of use of cortisone and other immunosuppressants in dermatology gives you an indication of how much of skin disease involves inflammation.

Inflammation occurs not only when bacteria or allergens are in the skin, but any time the immune system is triggered to react. The immune system of the body is made up of many different components that operate in different ways according to the targets and the conditions involved.

Let's look at the immune system of our body through the perspective of the defense system of a country. Like the defense forces of a country, there are different branches and different specialty qualifications of soldiers. Each group communicates with others to some degree, to mount an attack on invaders of different origin. Usually, these attacks are for the good of the individual/country, but sometimes these attacks persist without any obvious benefit. Instead, they produce destructive inflammation appearing as skin disease.

First, there is a network of sentries and early warning systems to check out potential invaders who do not seem to belong. When these sentries capture a foreign invader, they bring the invaders back to be checked out in "headquarters" by the lymphocytes (a specialized group of white blood cells) in the lymph nodes that drain their region. In the immune system, sentries include amoeba-like cells that gobble up bacteria and suspicious chemicals and "present" them to the lymphocytes to determine if action should be taken against them. In the skin, there is a highly specialized network of cells with long tendrils (known as Langerhans cells) that pick up suspicious chemicals and invaders, change shape, and then bring the suspects to present them to the lymphocytes in local lymph nodes where they can be evaluated. Foreign chemicals and debris recognized by the immune system are called "antigens." The technical name for both of these types of sentinels is "professional antigen presenting cells."

You may be wondering what is so special about these professional antigen presenting cells that gets them such a fancy name, and what they have to do with understanding why you have a rash. The foreign material or antigen picked up by these cells is presented to your immune system along with the "identity papers" of the presenting cells; both the characteristics of the presenting cells and the antigen are needed to see if your immune system is going to react. It's as if a key could not open a door unless the hand holding the key is also recognized. In this analogy, some part of the hand, such as the little finger, is part of what pushes the pins in the cylinder along with the ridges on the key, to open the lock. It's also similar to some modern car ignition keys, that not only have the specific pattern of ridges to turn on the ignition switch, but also have computer chip that must be recognized at the same time for the key to be recognized and the car to start.

This explains why one person may be allergic to a particular food or substance—milk, for example—and another person has no problem with the same substance. One reason is that different people's immune cells see the milk differently. The identity papers of the presenting cells create your own rather unique transplantation antigens, such as the ones that must be matched to prevent a transplanted kidney from being rejected. Kind of like your own hand holding the key. The need to recognize that whole complex of "you" plus the foreign antigen begins to explain why many conditions with inflammation of the skin can have different causes in different people.

Determining the Cause

Let's go back to the red-hot leg in the tent. How can we tell what is causing the problem? First, we take a history. Was poison ivy seen and touched on the first day in the woods? It usually takes two days for a poison ivy rash to erupt, so we have to have a possible or known contact with this plant around that time. Perhaps it was another plant that was the culprit, but that possibility would depend on where in the country the hiking occurred. Are there characteristic blisters in lines, as is often seen where poison ivy leaves brush against your skin? Is there a fever and tenderness, as might be seen in a bacterial infection called cellulitis? Are there large hives on the leg? We begin to explore different causes, each of which involves different branches of the immune system.

That takes us back to the defense system model. If it is poison ivy, which is a delayed hypersensitivity reaction, there will be lymphocytes invading the area and sending signals to call the attack. If it is a bacterial infection, another type of white cell called Polymorphonuclear leukocytes (PMNs) or "granulocytes" may be carrying out the attack against the bacteria involved. If it is hives, then a circulating "defense agent" called an antibody is most likely involved. And that would most likely be a specific antibody called IgE, which is involved in allergies to dust and pollen. What makes one skin rash different from the others is not only what branch of the body's defense system is attacking, but the vigor and the triggered response tendency of the target being attacked. The nature of the signals and the other "troops" brought into the battle also contribute to the unique rash, as do the other tendencies of the skin to behave to the signals and attacks. With hives, there is a release of histamine causing fluid to leave the blood vessels causing swelling. People with psoriasis have skin with a tendency to grow superfast with inflammatory stimuli.

When a disease-causing bacterium such as staph invades the skin, the body responds by rapidly building and deploying an army of defense agents that are specifically designed to attack and destroy the Staph. Those agents are antibodies, produced by a type of white cell called a plasma cell. Antibodies are large molecules that have a large "trap" or receptor at one end that holds onto some specific part of the bacteria or other target involved. Think of antibodies as a kind of heat-seeking missile, specifically designed and built to destroy one very specific target that has recently been identified as a major invading force. Once these have been deployed, they will act against that specific target (or one which looks very similar) very quickly. Some antibody responses, such as the ones that cause hives, pollen reactions, and even anaphylactic reactions with swelling and closure of the throat and airways, happen in a matter of minutes or seconds after breathing or eating the allergen involved. Other defense cells such as granulocytes are often part of the defense against invading bacteria. Granulocytes are loaded with little sacs of enzymes and antibacterial chemicals similar to peroxide, which can be dumped into the area or combined with the engulfed organisms to destroy bacteria and break down debris. Once they get their orders, they exit the blood vessels in the infected area in less than an hour. There they accumulate to engage the invaders and form the white accumulation we call "pus."

Lymphocytes have a very different method of working against what they see as the enemy. Lymphocytes are typically key soldiers in the attack against invaders inside our cells, including viruses, fungi, and the subtle changes which occur in tumors. They often act more like the detectives and the officers, deciding what needs to be attacked and starting the sequence of responses that sets off the attack. It's as if they need to do some reconnaissance and re-evaluation before they plan and carry out their attack. In the classic immunology I learned four to five decades ago, lymphocytes were part of the delayed hypersensitivity response. That response typically occurred 48 hours after contact with the allergen. For example, poison ivy contact rash is one such familiar reaction, usually occurring two days after contact with the plant.

Interested in science and research and headed for medical school, I was given an opportunity to volunteer in a nearby cancer research laboratory called Sloane Kettering in Rye, NY. Most of their studies at the time involved trying every sample they could find to see if the sample would kill cancer cells in culture. But in one small lab room that I got to visit after summer work as a lifeguard, scientists were studying how the immune response controlled cancer. Dr. Lloyd Old, who ran that lab, is now regarded as the father of tumor immunology. All the subsequent laboratories in which I did research revolved around this same crucial branch of the defense system, delayed hypersensitivity.

The Evolution of Immunology

Over the years, there have been numerous key strides in understanding the immune system and how it works. It is exciting to me to have been part of this work. It is also confidence-inspiring that the combination of my intellect and intuition concerning the fundamentals of the workings of the immune system, have led me to concepts, mentors, and research that, decades later, have repeatedly proven to be part of the future of immunology.

In the late 1800s, Robert Koch discovered the tuberculosis bacteria, and demonstrated that the killed bacteria, injected under the skin, caused a delayed swelling and inflammation in the skin of patients exposed to TB. It wasn't until 60 years later that Dr. Karl Landsteiner and Dr. Merrill Chase demonstrated that this reaction could be transferred by white blood cells, but not by serum alone (which contained the antibodies). Thus this form of immune reaction became known as cellular immunity (because it was carried by cells) or delayed hypersensitivity (because it manifested two days after exposure). Their studies ended the debate regarding whether immune cells or antibodies in the serum (humours) caused immunity. It showed that both played a role, and that both the feuding scientific groups were right.

Understanding of delayed hypersensitivity grew logarithmically through the time of my studies from the 1960s to 1980, and ever since then. As a result of a detailed biochemical understanding of the steps involved in the lymphocyte attack, a whole new class of targeted-lymphocyte-response inhibitors, known as the "biologics," is now being developed by pharmaceutical companies.

You may be familiar with the tuberculin tests on the forearm that are still done to this day to look for a delayed hypersensitivity indicating an exposure to or ongoing infection with tuberculosis. Delayed hypersensitivity is the main body defense system against not only certain bacterial infections that get inside the cells, but also against other more subtle invaders such as viruses, fungus, and tumors. All of these invaders require special detective work, because they tend to hide inside the body's cells, and not show all of their characteristics or antigens to the blood flowing by. They need a more clever intelligence branch of the defense system to ferret them out and initiate their destruction. Certain chemicals, both from plants and from man-made synthesis, can also incite delayed hypersensitivity. Poison ivy is one such plant that causes a rash on the skin because of the potent immune sensitizer chemicals it contains.

Most common tests for allergies are tests for specific antibodies in the blood. The tests for immediate allergies to substances we inhale from the air such as pollen and dust are typically measuring the reactions of particular types of antibodies, such as immunoglobulin E (IgE) to the allergen. IgE typically causes immediate reactions in hay fever, asthma, hives, and the potentially life-threatening anaphylactic reactions. Other classes of antibodies are measured to determine if there are specific antibodies to invading organisms as an indication that the infection is or was present at some time in the past. These include IgM, which is a first responder indicating recent disease, and IgG, indicating more past exposure and ongoing immune memory. IgA is the predominant antibody protecting mucous membranes in the digestive system.

You may be beginning to wonder why you should understand these differences in the body's defense system as much as you understand the differences in a country's defense system. The reason is that different branches of the immune system rule in the inflammation of different skin conditions. It is important to understand this when trying to understand both the triggers for the reaction and the timing of those triggers before the rash occurred.

But there is another big reason, poorly appreciated by physicians and even allergists. You need to understand what branch of the immune system is playing the leading role in a skin disorder to let you know what kind of laboratory test will give you the best information on the cause of the allergy/inflammation in the first place. In the armed forces model, you would not check out the army to find out what the navy was attacking. True, there is coordination among the different branches of the defense forces as there is in the immune system, but the best information comes from finding out the mission of the branch of the defense system involved.

So when an allergist does antibody tests for inhalant allergies to pollen, dust, and mold, they are likely to be predictive of the culprit causing immediate reactions such as asthma. But they are much less predictive of food allergies or skin reactions that involve lymphocytes and delayed hypersensitivity such as contact sensitivity, psoriasis, acne, or wart rejection. Dermatology may not have all the answers regarding disease causes, but extensive evaluation of what is going on under the skin by looking at biopsy samples under the microscope shows a lot about what types of cells are involved in the development of different types of skin lesions. Immune studies on different inflammatory skin diseases have expanded this knowledge further. If you have a puzzling skin problem, you may have gained information from both a biopsy and immune testing.

You can identify the cells of the main branch of the immune defense system involved in the attack from looking at a piece of skin tissue from the rash under the microscope. It makes most sense to do testing to find out what foods, chemicals, or microorganisms are triggering that attack by doing a test on the same type of cells that are involved in the rash. Tests on serum, the liquid part of the blood that contains the antibodies, have always been much easier to do than tests on the cells, so the majority of testing still is like asking the Navy what the Air Force is doing. That is why choosing the best form of testing can be very helpful in getting a relevant answer to what is causing the problem.

Factors Influencing Reactivity

If people we know come into our community, we usually welcome them with open arms. If we don't recognize them, however, or if there were suddenly a small noticeable group of suspicious-looking people around, we would probably not tolerate their presence. But if this group grew gradually and became part of the community, we would become used to them.

The concept of tolerance also exits in the immune system. Classically, it depends on the dose and the route of entry of the foreign "antigen," and what signals or chemicals accompany it. When there are large amounts of a given material around, the system is said to be in high-dose tolerance and there is no reactivity against it. Tolerance can also be induced by very small, almost homeopathic doses of a substance. Intermediate amounts of the invader can stimulate reactivity against it. You can see that changing the level of presence of a foreign inhabitant in our body (such as yeast or bacteria in the intestines) could change the reactivity to it. We now know that these changes in reactivity are accompanied by changes in the chemical signals sent by the immune system. We also know that there are different parts of our genetic code that open up or close to either send those signals, compensate for the challenge going on, or shut down when a challenge is removed. The changes in these compensations and signals may account for changes sometimes known as a "detox reaction," that occur when a harmful organism is destroyed in one's body. *(see Tolerance figure on page 153)*

Structure

Just as sentries might bring back the first invading spies to central headquarters for questioning, the immune presenting cells bring back to the lymph nodes the samples captured. Those are the nodes that get big and possibly tender when you have an infection in an area, such as in your upper neck during a sore throat. Sentries and other types of white blood cells from the area of disturbance are carried to the lymph nodes along channels called lymphatics. The lymph nodes also recruit more white cells to act as a defense force against the specific culprits spotted in the disturbance occurs. That is why they get swollen and enlarged when there is an infection or allergy going on. In that enlargement, the branch of the immune system necessary for the attack is chosen and expanded. This might involve either an increase in plasma cells producing an antibody against a specific bacterium, or a buildup of lymphocytes that recognize a particular allergen, virus, or marker on tumor cells.

In our world, defense systems begin on the local level, and do not necessarily involve the armed services. Our houses have fences, locks on the doors, watchful neighbors, and/or alarm systems that notify police and neighbors of a breach in security. The same is true of the skin, where local defenses also play an important role in the overall immune defense process. One of the most basic local forms of defense is having a barrier relatively impermeable to liquids and bacteria. When this is broken in conditions such as eczema, or destroyed by scratching, bacteria and allergens can get into the skin. Skin cells give off antibacterial substances to fight local infection. Cells in the skin also send information signals to the immune system.

Just as with the armed services, messages are sent among various branches of the defense forces to recruit or reverse help. The immune cells send chemical signals called "cytokines" to transmit signals to other parts of the immune system.

More of My Journey

Back in medical school, in 1968, I worked with Dr. Barry R. Bloom at Albert Einstein, trying to isolate one of the first such information molecules to be identified. It was called Migration Inhibitory Factor (MIF), and it was a chemical signal from lymphocytes that caused the macrophages (white blood cells) to stop moving and collect around an area where lymphocytes detected a foreign chemical from an infection. I collected blood from TB patients at Bellevue, separated out the lymphocytes, and grew them in culture plates with or without an extract of tuberculosis bacteria (tuberculin). Inside those cultures, I placed a tiny capillary tube packed with macrophages, which could spill out the open end. We found that the macrophages tended to cluster around the mouth of the capillary tube in a small circle (that is, not migrate) when the TB patient lymphocytes had tuberculin in the culture. Since that early experiment, more than fifty lymphocyte signal molecules have been identified and named, in addition to many other types of immune communication molecules. Each of these not only regulates the system, but is also a potential target for disruption of the immune system in a way that could cause inflammation and skin rash.

ALAN M DATTNER, MD

We have gone from seeing the immune system working in a linear sequence as a row of dominos, to seeing a whole interacting network of effects back and forth among multiple signaling "troops." The entire field of "biologics" to suppress immune reactions such as those in psoriasis or rheumatoid arthritis has been built on targeting the signal molecules from the immune system. Dr. Bloom, with his vast knowledge and broad perspective on health, went on to be the head of the prestigious Harvard School of Public Health.

From eczema to psoriasis to acne to more uncommon skin rashes, inflammation is a big part of the reason the disorder is active. We have no problem understanding why there is inflammation in a Staph infection or even in hives, but in other disorders, the reason is less apparent. In psoriasis, early drugs such as corticosteroids and cell division inhibitors (for instance, methotrexate) that were sometimes used for cancer, all inhibit the inflammatory attack of lymphocytes in the skin. The newer highly-targeted drugs called "biologics" inhibit specific steps in the cellular immune attack. They sometimes shut down the inflammation and rash in psoriasis, but on occasion shut down the defense against tuberculosis and lymphomas. There is often evidence of an attack, such as white blood cells of various types seen when the skin is examined under a microscope in that condition. There may even be evidence of one's own chemical soldiers, with antibodies visible by special studies, right at the microscopic area where the damage occurs.

If the immune system attack is the cause of a skin disorder, the next question is what part of the defense system is attacking, what is the exact target, and why is this attack happening? What is it that set the defense forces looking for that target in the first place? Was there some microorganism, chemical, or food that was riling up the immune system that looked very much like what was being targeted and attacked in the skin? In the past, we had some tools to examine that question. We could look at the antibodies in the blood and see what they were directed at, see the address in their program, see exactly what they bound onto. If the target they were directed against was a yeast, we could see if other types of yeasts also bound to that same antibody. We could compare the address of other targets to see if the missile that was directed against some allergen or food or bacterial product, might also be directed against the target in the skin being attacked. Here we had a potential way to examine the blood and find out what was setting off an inflammatory skin rash.

Unfortunately, there was a problem here. Once again, you could not examine missiles from the Air Force to understand what the Navy was doing. We can assume an overlap in purpose, but that is just an assumption. The problem is that the attack from the immune system in many skin diseases most importantly involves lymphocytes in a cellular immune attack. So comparing skin targets versus various environmental targets for antibodies doesn't necessarily give any good information about what the target was.

We needed a way to compare the response of human white blood cells to various targets to see if the spectrum of what they were recognizing and directed against could explain why a particular environmental stimulus could lead to a specific attack leading to a skin disease such as acne, eczema, or psoriasis. Together with Dr. William Levis, we created a test-tube laboratory system to ask that very question.

Our Breakthrough Discovery Opening Holistic Dermatology

According to Dermatology textbooks, the cause of most inflammatory skin diseases is not known. Often, there is a very specific kind of attack by particular branches of the immune system in a given skin disease, such as acne. Various environmental exposures, microbes, and foods have been linked to specific cases of various skin conditions, but those same exposures did not necessarily cause the same condition in others. Based on the underlying assumption that a disease was an entity, a distinct "thing," it was believed that that entity should have a single cause. There was no way to explain why different individuals with the same disease would have different causes, so the apparent cause of an inflammatory skin disease by different agents in different people was dismissed as "anecdotal." The reason that much of dermatology treatment has been suppression of inflammatory reactions is based on this conviction that we cannot know what stimulus set off the rash, and that it was the same stimulus for each patient.

From Californians interested in natural health during the late 1960s, I had heard about foods as vital in causing and curing diseases but had no way to explain these reported observations scientifically. I had been in five different cellular immunology laboratories by the time that I completed my dermatology training, in each case with brilliant preceptors; but those years had produced limited cutting edge discoveries and publications of my own. During this time, I had been back and forth between research and clinical medicine in medical school, internship, residency, and fellowship. Each year of working with patients deepened both my understanding and questioning of how the cellular immune system could be triggered to cause the illnesses I was seeing. I then joined Dr. William Levis at the Dermatology Branch of the National Cancer Institute (NCI) as a visiting Scientist in his laboratory. Together, Bill and I had over 25 years of cellular immunology between us, which was likely more than any other dermatology team in the world at that time.

Our research at the NCI completely opened up my understanding of the previous dilemma and the path to understanding the cause of inflammatory skin disorders. Let me share what our studies revealed in the context of the defense model above. A rash with underlying inflammation, such as eczema, often involves a very specific target in the skin. White blood cells specifically find that target, move into the area, and attack. We knew that lymphocytes were part of the attacking forces seen in biopsies of the rash in a number of skin diseases including acne, eczema, and psoriasis. What would make them attack a specific layer of the skin or even a specific molecular structure? In uncommon blistering diseases such as pemphigus, antibodies can be identified along the line at which the skin layers separate. Further studies have shown that, in pemphigus, those antibodies target the very spots where skin cells attach to each other. But in other disorders, it is the white cells and not the antibodies that seem to play the biggest role in the attack. How could they be set off by a food or other environmental exposure? What might those environmental triggers for the immune attack be?

I will try to describe the experimental laboratory studies we created to ask that question.

We knew that we could separate out white blood cells containing lymphocytes from people sensitive to a particular bacterial product such as tuberculin, then add tuberculin to the cells' environment and see them respond by dividing and making more lymphocytes. We presumed that those new lymphocytes were specifically sensitive to the original stimulus, but we had no proof. We could also get them to respond to a chemical called "DNCB" (DiNitroChloroBenzene) that caused a delayed, blistery skin rash, similar to poison ivy. The first question we wanted to ask was whether lymphocytes stimulated by DNCB all had specific receptors for DNCB, or whether they would also have receptors for the tuberculin to which the blood donor was responsive.

To ask that question, we placed white blood cells from a human blood donor volunteer (allergic to both allergens) into a flask with culture medium and added either a little of the tuberculin extract or DNCB, and allowed the cells to be stimulated to grow in response to the specific allergen and grow in an incubator. We then took out the cells, and put them into little wells with either tuberculin or

DNCB. They responded only to the original stimulating allergen, and not to the other one that was not used. Later, we showed that if we used stimulating cells from another donor to "present" the allergen, there was no stimulation unless the other donor shared transplantation antigens with the original donor. Furthermore, the greater the similarity of the transplantation antigens of the " antigen presenter" white cells to those of the original presenter, the greater the response using the same antigen. We had shown that the genetically determined transplantation antigens controlled the immune response. That was the essence of what Dr. Baruj Benacerraf was honored for as one of three recipients of the Nobel Prize in Medicine in 1980. More important to me was that we showed that similar transplantation plus foreign antigen complexes gave strong responses. This ability of similar stimuli to incite a similar response is known as "cross-reactivity" (*see cross-reaction illustration on page 57*).

So there must either be substances that deposit in the skin to serve as targets, or the actual structures, chemicals or inhabitants in the skin look similar to external targets that set off the immune soldiers to attack anything that looks similar. Furthermore, the target is unique to the individual, because it contains the presenting aspect that has characteristics (transplantation antigens) unique to that individual. Suddenly, I had an outpouring of data that explained why eggs can set off eczema in one person and not in another. I use the word outpouring because we got confirmatory data about these cross-reactive relationships in multiple studies, with samples run in triplicate, at several different concentrations, rolling off the radiation counter (which measures the division of white blood cells) once or twice a week for more than two years. We published several articles, and were among the first to show this relationship using human lymphocytes. I was a rising star, and was offered several academic positions to pursue my studies (I mention this only to illustrate how cutting edge our studies were). The validity and applicability of our discoveries on cross-reactivity in disease was confirmed by a growing body of published data, and by a second Nobel prize to Doherty and Zinkernagel for related studies, in 1996.

Poignantly, more than 20 years later, in the last issue of the 20th century, an article in the prestigious *New England Journal of Medicine* discussed specific instances in which cross-reactive attack initiated by specific organisms led to specific diseases in humans. Studies since then have identified the sequence of five or so amino acids that are exactly the same in the protein of the organism and the protein of the organ being attacked (*see immune recognition diagram page 57*).

It was my early glimpse of the nature of this cross-reactivity, or molecular mimicry, as it is known now (more on this later in the book), that validated the ideas that foods and environmental insults could initiate skin diseases. Equipped with that perspective, two decades before it became known in the medical community, I began combing my patients' experience and history during the time preceding their rash onset for possible triggers. I later combined that questioning with the perspective that came from what was later named Functional Medicine, seeking conditions that would allow those food aggravators to escape into the circulation to cause trouble. More than anything else, these studies gave me the certainty that there were precipitating causes for inflammatory attacks on the skin that could be found and even reversed, allowing the skin diseases to heal at the level of cause, rather than by suppression.

Since that time, there have been progressions of scientific studies on a myriad of immune system pathways, functional medicine relationships, and other factors that have enriched and complicated my understanding of immunity and inflammation. One very surprising area in immunology, which I learned about nearly two decades after my formal studies, was a branch of the immune system that offered an entire new set of ways we could potentially have inflammatory informational signals from something we ate or encountered. I practically had to be sitting down to absorb this information. This is now referred to as the "innate" immune system or the Toll-Like Receptors (TLRs). These TLRs are not only present in other animals; they are present in invertebrates such **as insects and even plants** and other forms of life. They are a very primitive immune system that warns us about the presence of different classes of foreign attackers. As does the sentry at the furthest outpost and the sailor atop the mast in the crow's nest, these TLRs offer the first warning of trouble ahead, and set in motion more sophisticated branches of our immune defense system. Just imagine that we might receive information from plants and other things we eat and touch that speak to our immune system in a way that sets off a reaction in our skin. This is a new area, and similar to many new areas on the horizon, has the potential to be explored for what it might tell us about how foods and environmental exposures could be triggering inflammation in the form of ordinary and unusual skin conditions.

A side note: in some cases of diseases with unknown causes, such as PLEVA for example, or lymphomatoid diseases, we have found hints of active viruses involved, or at least elevated anti-virus antibody levels. This suggests that some form for continuation of infection or reactivation of viruses is contributing to the disorder. In those cases, in addition to my usual program of fixing the "leaky gut" issues, I have used various substances to gain better control of the viruses. This includes both enhancing the immune system, and using a variety of natural substances which have general and specific antiviral properties. Some of these substances have been discussed, others are known, and still others are proprietary and are still being developed.

Some of these have already proven to be effective in patients with autoimmune disorders associated with elevated viral titers. Working with a health professional is the best practice to address such cases.

Illustration

Immune recognition and cross-reactive immune recognition

How does the immune system find and attack the right "bad guys"? The first frame shows the T-lymphocytes (white blood cells) recognizing the foreign "antigen" with their receptors. Those T-cells divide and create a population with the same receptors, which then search all over the body for similar targets. If some part of your skin cells or altered skin cells happen to have a similar appearance, those specifically sensitized cells will attack that skin and cause an allergic or autoimmune "cross-reactive" response.

Immune Recognition

Lymphocytes recognize foreign microbes or harmful substances or threats from within (tumors, infected cells), then divide to form an army of lymphocytes that recognize the specific threat to attack and destroy it.

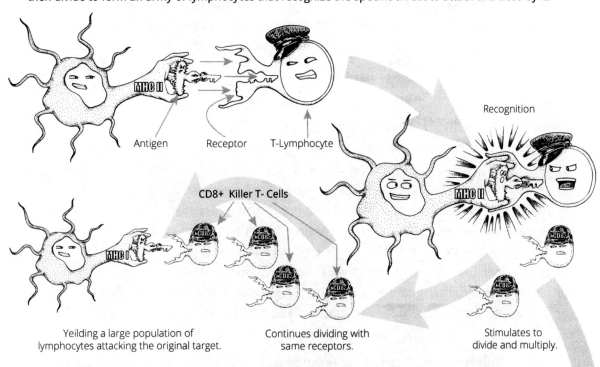

Antigen   Receptor   T-Lymphocyte

Recognition

CD8+ Killer T- Cells

Yeilding a large population of lymphocytes attacking the original target.

Continues dividing with same receptors.

Stimulates to divide and multiply.

Cross-reactive Immune Recognition

Similar looking substances (by molecular mimicry) may be recognized as harmful targets in a process known as cross-reaction. If one of those cross-reactive substances is part of your body, there may be inflammation from an auto-immune attack.

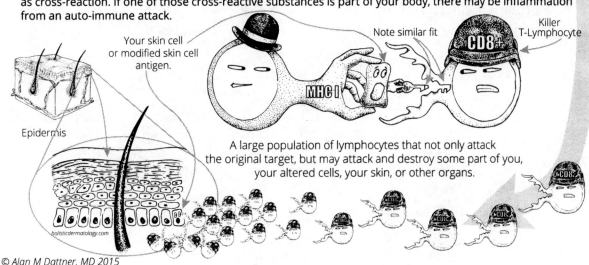

Your skin cell or modified skin cell antigen.

Note similar fit

Killer T-Lymphocyte

Epidermis

A large population of lymphocytes that not only attack the original target, but may attack and destroy some part of you, your altered cells, your skin, or other organs.

holisticdermatology.com

Summary

The body's immune defense system plays a key role in most skin conditions, and especially in those that are red or itchy. Understanding how the immune system works gives us an opportunity to explore and modify the underlying network of causes that lead to the battle of inflammation going on in our skin and body. The more understanding that you and your healing team have of your defense system and the different branches involved, the better you can interpret data from your experience, diagnosis, biopsy, lab results, and other sources. The strategy you develop from this understanding as it applies to dietary, infectious, environmental, genetic, and emotional aggravators in your own life affecting your skin can help you avoid or reduce the reliance on immunosuppressive medications. Prolonged use of immunosuppressive medications can lead to a buildup of local and systemic side effects that disfigure the skin, reduce normal function, or even reduce active longevity. Active inflammation in the skin, and the underlying digestive, environmental, and hormonal disturbances, often affect other organs of the body. So using your skin condition as a warning sign offers a way to improve not only your appearance but also your health and vitality. Using a more natural approach to correct the underlying causes of skin disease, governed by a working understanding of how the immune system functions, is the best tactic for maintaining healthy skin and a healthy body.

Inflammation does not come out of nowhere, but has a network of causes. In many cases, the cause is stimulation by external and internal triggers. Identifying and avoiding those triggers, correcting the process that allows those triggers access, and fixing other paths by which they contribute to disease, is a key method in turning off inflammatory disorders of the skin.

CHAPTER 5
HERBAL TREATMENTS

When I was a teenager, I read a story in the newspaper about a couple in New Jersey who picked wild mushrooms and ate them at their barbecue. Unfortunately, the mushrooms turned out to be poisonous, and they began getting sick with liver failure. I read that they sent to Germany for the cure. I'm not sure if they received the cure in time. More than three decades later, I learned that the cure they likely sent for was a purified herbal product named Legalon, derived from the common plant milk thistle. At that time, we had nothing in current Western medical practice to help a damaged liver, yet there was a well-respected herbal product in Europe for this purpose. The herb was growing wild in fields and along roadsides in the United States, and its uses to support the liver were well known to herbalists. Medicine in that era had "purified" itself with science and branched off from the herbal traditions from which it originated, and had left behind a world of potential treatments for a multitude of conditions. Herbal medicine was considered to be somewhere between quackery and witchcraft.

Times have changed. Savvy scientists have tested the active ingredient in milk thistle, namely silymarin, and shown it to have activity in protecting against liver disease and healing liver cells in a variety of ways. A look at Pub Med (an online database from the National Library of Medicine of all of the peer-reviewed scientific medical studies published in medical journals) shows more than 2375 references to scientific studies on silymarin, many of which point to silymarin protecting the liver of both animals and humans. Many of the studies show how this protection occurs at the cellular level. This is just one example of how herbs offer treatments of conditions for which there are no existing traditional drug treatments.

Many commonly used herbs and their crude extracts have the benefit of having much greater margins of safety than pharmaceuticals. A constant influx of new herbs into the care of skin conditions has occurred over the past several years, from folk usage, other traditions, and new discoveries based on scientific studies.

Combinations of herbs allow balancing of numerous factors. Herbs are generally closer to foods than to drugs, so that their margin of safety is greater. That makes it much more sensible to try the safer herbs when suspecting a condition about which you are not yet certain. For example, using dandelion root tea to support the liver when one suspects insufficient breakdown of products in that organ makes more sense than experimenting with a drug strong enough to stop the rash that is probably occurring because of poor liver function.

Herbs provide a time-tested therapeutic alternative for skin disorders, with several major advantages in the right situations. Evidence of herb use, and the patterns of use, has been passed down in cultures as folk medicine for thousands of years. This means that at a primitive observational level, there is a lot of experience with the effects of these herbs in healing. Complex systems of matching the right herbal combination to the individual with an illness have developed in older cultures, and we can use some of the wisdom of these systems in our choice of herbs today. For some people, that may mean going to, for instance, an American or Chinese Herbalist or an Ayurvedic practitioner. In any case, the most effective herb or herb combination chosen usually addresses more than one characteristic of the ailing person. For example, berberine from bearberry or goldenseal is bitter, and considered "cooling" so it may be selected to kill bacteria in someone who has evidence of "heat" in the digestive system. Heat in the digestive system could be loosely described as over-activity producing increased blood flow to that organ system. Berberine would, on the other hand, best be avoided in someone with a cool, underactive digestive system.

To offer the best possible care, use of herbal healing traditions *must also* respect the principles of good conventional medicine. For example, a formula of Tea Tree oil for a fungal condition is just not a good idea in a patient who has an allergic contact sensitivity to essential oils, as it will cause that patient to break out in a rash.

Similarly, comfrey has amazing properties for healing small cuts and wounds. But there are two cautions here. It works so well that, in an improperly cleaned wound, it can cause the skin to heal over grit and foreign materials not properly cleansed out of the wound. I have seen such a healed wound break down repeatedly as a result of foreign material caught deep in the skin. The other caution is that comfrey contains pyrrolizidine alkaloids that are potentially hepatotoxic (toxic to the liver) and carcinogenic, so most herbalists would not use it in large quantities on extensive skin wounds, and there is some controversy regarding its use internally.

How Herbs are Related to Us, and Why They Make Sense

Plants need to perform many of the same functions that we do. Since they often spend the whole day in the sun, they need to protect themselves from being burned. Burning is an "oxidation" reaction, like the browning of paper or the rusting of iron. The energy absorbed that is not handled by green chlorophyll has to be quieted or "quenched." Plants have systems of antioxidants to do this. Vitamin C is one of those antioxidants most of us are familiar with. But plants also have more complex molecules such as bioflavonoids (found in yellow plants), or carotene family products (found in orange and red plants) to share the job of quenching the sun's energy. All of these work together in the plant to keep it from getting damaged by oxidation from the sun. For that reason, using a crude extract rather than a purified single component of an herb makes sense. That way you get the whole antioxidant system that the plant used.

Another reason herbs make sense is that they have been used successfully for many generations. Valuable observations have been passed down over many lifetimes. The collection of this lore into various traditions of herbal healing offers a goldmine of potential treatments.

New observations in the fields of genetics and immunology offer an additional perspective on why plant medicines have the potential for being so helpful. Plants not only have to perform similar functions to ours, but even share with us some of the same molecular machinery to do so. For example, identifying and repelling foreign invaders has recently been shown to be initiated by a primitive branch of our immune system known as the "innate" or inborn system. The amazing discovery is that our innate system resembles the defense system found in all sorts of other life forms, including insects and plants! Imagine that. Our system has some of the same molecular receptors to detect danger as do the plants. No wonder plants and their extracts have an ability to help us fend off disease. And this is only one of the reasons plants can be helpful.

Plants have also evolved the ability to ward off specific predators, infections, and tumors, and to deal with stresses unique to the locale in which they grow. Since plants cannot move to get away from danger, they have the ability to increase production of certain protective chemicals when they are under attack; the specific chemicals they produce is a direct result of the specific stressor they are facing. Sometimes these chemicals are offensive to humans, as in the smell of tomato stems, which repel certain pests. Some plants will make defensive chemicals only under various conditions—such as when they're being attacked—that they don't make normally. Anti-cancer activity observed in particular plants that could not be reproduced in scientific trials may have been resulted from a response to particular organisms attacking those plants. And sometimes it is these protective or stress-induced chemicals that account for the medicinal properties of the herbs. This is one of the reasons that a particular species of plant may provide healing in one situation, and not be helpful in another. Production of compounds called salvestrols by the immune system of plants to ward off pests and disease are an example of this. These salvestrols act on an enzyme called CYP1B1 present only in cancer cells causing the cancer cells, but not the normal cells, to commit suicide. Unfortunately, plants grown with pesticides do not need to produce these compounds to protect themselves, so the majority of our crops have lower amounts of these important substances.

Methods of extraction of medicinal ingredients from plants have evolved according to herbal tradition, and vary according to the plant and sometimes even the condition being treated. Some active components dissolve in alcohol while others are best extracted with water. Good herbalists and good herbal companies may have better products because they identify the herbs used more carefully, perform extraction better, concentrate their product with more active ingredient and less fiber, stabilize the preparation, and check for the presence of active ingredients with modern technologic methods.

Each species of plant that has been studied has been found to contain dozens if not hundreds of different chemical ingredients, many of which have potential activity in humans. A list of all of the identified chemical parts of an herb, still can only give a hint of what that herb can do. We can be safe in guessing that many of these components worked together synergistically for the plant to survive and thrive. So it would not be a big jump of faith to guess that these different components would also work together synergistically when ingested or used as a topical by people to heal their ailments. That is the belief of herbalists, who feel that relatively crude extracts are more effective than purified products. This differs from the philosophy of pharmacologists and pharmaceutical manufacturers, who prefer to isolate only the most active compounds and use those for their stronger effects. I believe that both philosophies have some merit, and that a relative enrichment for active ingredients may be the wisest method. Both an understanding of the science involving detailed studies of specific extracted chemicals, and the lore from other traditions, which brings observation over many generations, can help guide best choices of herbal treatment among a myriad of possibilities. Individual plant extracts used as herbs contain complex mixtures of active chemicals, and have many effects. I have used some herbs for years, only to hear of another herbalist who has used the same herb for a very different purpose.

It is beyond the scope of this book to describe all of the herbs used for the skin. If I devoted a lifetime to the task, I would still be finding new information as I tried to write about the old. And there are simply not enough pages in this book to do justice to the subject (one of my herbal teachers, David Winston, once told me he had over 300 linear feet of herbal books on the shelves in his library. Much in those books probably relates to skin, and I'm sure his library has grown since). What I will do is describe a few of the herbs that I use in my practice. Some are widely available commercially, and others are available in specific geographic locales. You may want to favor the herbs that are available locally for your treatment, both for best price and best product. What is most important here is to gain some perspective on the power of herbs in disease, the different perspectives used for choosing them and combining them, and how they weave in and out of scientific medicine over the years.

Various traditions have developed a code of the primary and secondary effects of herbs from observations over the years. That simplifies our understanding of when and how to choose them; for instance which digestive herbs to use for a given person in a given circumstance. Decisions are based on knowing what the herb does, and what is likely to be going on in the person who is ill. For example, if someone is irritated by food going through their esophagus and digestive system, an herb that coats the mucus membranes would make the most sense to use. So you might choose marshmallow root tea or deglycyrrhizinated licorice before eating to coat the delicate lining of the digestive system.

Most herbal traditions, Western and otherwise, attempt to treat the underlying causes of skin diseases as they are understood by that tradition. So herbs actually used often address the organs of digestion (stomach and intestines) and elimination (liver and kidneys) rather than the skin itself. Below is a list of herbs used directly on or for the skin itself. This is a brief summary, rather than a definitive guide to the identification and use of these plants.

Some herbs that are commonly used on the skin include:

- **Witch Hazel**: used for minor scratches, bites, swellings, and wounds to soothe the affected area. It has astringent properties, which constricts swollen tissue and small vessels that might be bleeding. This also makes it useful for swollen and varicose veins of the skin.

- **Chamomile**: applied as a cream or tincture for its mild antiseptic and anti-inflammatory properties. Tinctures are useful in the mouth for sores of the mucus membranes

- **Chickweed**: helpful for its mild anti-inflammatory properties infused in a cream or ointment; may be helpful for mild eczema as an ointment. This can be very helpful in stepping down from using topical cortisone cream when more anti-inflammatory activity than what is found in a bland cream is needed.

- **Plantain**: a commonly found plant in lawns or walked-on areas that is very helpful for calming down stings or insect bites. The leaves are picked, washed if possible, crushed or chewed, and placed as a poultice over the bite or sting. This is a very important plant to know, because it can usually be found out-doors wherever stinging and biting insects are found.

- **Jewelweed**: a plant with a translucent, water-containing stem, often found in wet areas, which can be helpful if crushed and applied to the area where poison ivy just touched the skin, to reduce the chances of poison ivy developing. Soap and water, the sooner the better, also helps in this prevention of skin outbreak two days hence.

- **Aloe vera**: the clear jell-like juice from the inside of this succulent plant is used as a remedy for soothing minor burns. The wisdom of keeping an aloe plant in the kitchen for first and second degree burns has been validated by medical studies. It has some beneficial effects for sunburn as well. Use the clear portion in the center of the leaves and avoid the yellow part just inside the green leaf itself. That part contains chemicals known as "anthraquinones" which have laxative and anti-psoriatic effects, but can cause rashes, sun sensitivity, and more.

- **Oats**: Oatmeal baths have been a mainstay of calming down itchy rashes in conventional dermatology and herbal treatment as well.

- **Berberine**: Present in herbs such as barberry, goldenseal, and Chinese gold-enthread. These are bitter and anti-microbial and can be used internally or topically to control superficial infections. They are nowhere near as powerful as antibiotics available today for serious infections.

- **Essential oils, such as Tea Tree and Oregano oil**: these have powerful anti-microbial effects and can be used to treat fungal infections of the skin, bacterial infections, and even acne in some cases. They must be diluted, and repeated exposure can lead to development of contact allergy to these products.

- **Stinging Nettle:** Fresh stinging nettle has tiny histamine-filled hairs that will cause stinging and a rash if they brush against your skin. But extracts of this plant have been helpful in calming down itchy rashes.

- **Calendula:** From marigolds, calendula has both mild anti-microbial and anti-inflammatory properties, so it can be helpful in mild skin irritation, applied topically. It can be applied to irritated skin and has been used in the past on skin ulcers.

Evaluating Herbal Products

Remember that just because a product contains herbs, which are natural ingredients, this inclusion does not, in itself, make the product harmless. Poison ivy is a natural plant, but you would be very careful to avoid touching it because of the rash it could cause. Herbs are also weeds, and you can become allergic to them from repeated use. Some of that repeated use can come from their presence in various natural products such as creams and shampoos where they have been included either for fragrance or healing properties. Some other herbs, including ones that are highly diluted so that they are safe to use in homeopathy, such as aconite, are highly toxic and dangerous in herbal form. Herbs that are incorporated into creams have a list of other components along with them. Sometimes, it is those other products that cause allergic or irritant reactions in certain people. So you must not only look for the herb that is useful in a cream, but also look for the ingredients that are either known to cause you trouble or are suspected of causing you trouble, and avoid those.

Adulteration of expensive herbs with lesser ones has been a problem occurring over and over since the beginning of history. Good herbal companies receive their herbs in whole form so that they can be identified by appearance, taste, and smell. They check for active ingredients by not only the feel and touch, but also with modern technology methods such as HPLC, High Pressure Liquid Chromatography, which is one method that helps identify exactly which components are present. DNA hybridization techniques have recently been used as the gold standard of herb product identification; this practice is not reliable because although the techniques are among the tools for identifying the plant itself, they are often not useful in identifying extracts, which do not contain the plant DNA. It is wise to either be able to identify characteristics of the herbal products you are using, or to use a company you trust, that is run by knowledgeable and ethical herbalists. I have been fortunate to meet and get to know many of the herbalists who run the companies that make the products I use in my practice.

Safety and Interactions

Most herbs have a gentler effect and much wider range of safety than drugs. You, or the person administering those herbs, should have knowledge of the degree, varieties of, and identification of potential toxicity. As with foods, allergic reactions are possible if you are already allergic to other members of the same botanical family. So this must always be kept in mind if you have strong or dangerous allergies. Essential oils have powerful anti-microbial effects, but they would be a poor choice if you already are allergic to one such as peppermint.

Herbs have traditionally been used in combination preparations in most traditions including Western herbalism, Chinese medicine, and Ayurvedic medicine. It should be reassuring to know that skillful combination according to traditional principles often results in fewer rather than more unwanted side effects. Individual differences of the "energetics" of the individual codified by each tradition, is important in choice. For example, if several different herbs are available to treat an infection of the skin, ones that are known to have a cooling energy would be chosen if the infected area were red, hot, and swollen. So, too, would be the internal and external nature of the illness being treated, whether it is an inflammation or an infection. Both the lore of herbal traditions and studies in medical science can help in the choice of herbs that most effective and least likely to cause harm in a particular skin disorder situation. Science would have us be aware of specific genetic differences, such as defective enzymes for breakdown of specific herbal components. Testing is becoming more available for specific defects involving inability to break down various drugs by the liver and other organs. After an adverse reaction to a specific drug, such defects in metabolism may be suspected and testing should be done to avoid similar reactions to other medications processed by the same chemical machinery.

Herbs, drugs, and foods can turn on, turn down, or compete with the liver and body's mechanism for breaking down and getting rid of other herbal or pharmaceutical components in the body. So it is very important to evaluate the possible interactions of herbs that you are about to add if you are using medications whose concentrations in your body are crucial to health or life. If the medication is preventing, for example, blood clots or rejection of a transplanted organ, you would not want that medication broken down faster so that the protection stopped. If the medication was effective in a very narrow concentration range and toxic above that concentration, you would not want to take an herb that slowed down breakdown, and raised the concentration to toxic levels. There is now substantial understanding of these interactions, such as the effect of grapefruit on the liver enzymes breaking down a whole family of drugs. Those drugs are made less active by a specific enzyme in the liver known as Cytochrome P450 3A4. Grapefruit juice inhibits this enzyme, causes slower breakdown and increased blood levels of those drugs, and the possible side effects from those higher levels. Similar understanding of the breakdown process of many other drugs and the foods and herbs that affect them is now in the medical literature. It makes sense to explore what is already known about interactions before beginning specific herbs if you are already on medications important to your health.

Your Family's Folk Medicine

Consider what herbs and herbal extracts you or your family already use as spices, remedies, or as the key ingredient from which your medicines have been made. Notice, too, the herbal components in creams, shampoos, toiletries, and cosmetics that you use.

Write out a list of your family's traditions of health. What did your grandmother's grandmother always say about taking care of a cold? About what to do with butter? About which plant would keep you strong and healthy? It might serve you well to give these "old-fashioned" remedies a try and add them to your arsenal of healthy practices. From there you can build on what you actually already know, and add other herbal products to keep your skin and body healthy. For example, you may have witch hazel in your medicine cabinet to apply to small scrapes. You might enjoy peppermint tea after a meal to help your digestion. If your family makes tomato sauce, the oregano, basil, thyme, garlic, and other spices you add for flavor are also powerful anti-microbial herbs that kill any mold in the tomatoes that are beginning to get soft and "turn" bad.

ALAN M DATTNER, MD

Using Herbs

As you can see, you are probably already using herbs, and you probably have some idea how you interact with a number of them. They clearly lie between food and drugs in both their potency and safety. As you extend your use of herbs, you need to learn about both the herbs' properties and how they work in relation to you. A skilled practitioner can help you greatly in this process, especially if you have health disorders to treat. Many herbs have both primary and secondary actions, so it is best to choose ones whose list of actions best match your needs and constitution.

Dosages depend on both the practitioner and patient. British herbalists tend to give teaspoon doses of herbal tinctures. Most bottles suggest dropper doses. One herbalist I know, Matthew Woods, uses herbal tinctures for their energetic qualities, much closer to homeopathy, so he chooses one-to-three-drop doses. Of course with homeopathy, small to infinitesimal doses are used. There are toxic herbs, so powerful that amounts greater than homeopathic doses could potentially be a danger to life. These toxic herbs should only be used by a practitioner skilled in their use, and even then, only with great respect.

Some individuals seem to need higher doses of herbs or medications to get an effect, while others seem to be very sensitive to every treatment. Taking this into account helps choose what range of dosage to explore by you or your practitioner to whom you communicate this information. A difficult condition may warrant a very gentle approach to avoid upsetting your system. A dangerous condition might also require aggressive action using either herbs to attempt to avoid the use of pharmaceuticals when possible, or pharmaceuticals when they are really necessary to avoid further harm or death to the patient. These choices should be made with a skilled practitioner who has an understanding of not only the herbs and the condition present, but also the medical alternatives and when to switch over to them or refer for their use. I recite these warnings because although they may seem obvious, quick and well-calculated decisions may need to be made with these considerations kept in mind.

Even with foods, it is important to know both the immediate and long-term dangers as well as benefits. It is all the more so true for herbs. There is wisdom in rotating the herbs you are using, just as one should do with foods, to avoid developing an allergy. Get the effect you are seeking, and then take a break when possible. New knowledge is developing clinically and in the laboratory on a constant basis, so it is helpful to review the literature about the herbal preparations you are taking to understand the effects on other organs in your body, especially if other symptoms or abnormal test results emerge.

In summary, there is a world of herbal treatments available, and with learning, guidance, and careful observation, these products can help your skin condition, either alone or combined with other forms of therapy.

CHAPTER 6

LIVER METABOLISM

Sometimes I hear a patient say, "I came here for my skin. What does my liver have to do with my skin?" Remember that the liver is one of the major organs involved in transforming problem and toxic chemicals in your bloodstream, and getting them out of your body. The skin also has a lesser role as a fallback for ridding the body of unwanted chemicals through the sweat ducts and oil glands. When the liver or kidneys are overwhelmed, the skin helps take over, by emitting allergenic and toxic materials onto its surface. Acne and other skin conditions may result from this process. Also, excess hormones such as estrogen are eliminated via the action of the liver. Problems with this function result in hormonal imbalances such as hormone-aggravated acne. As you understand the role of the liver in removing and breaking down all kinds of chemicals and fragments in the blood, you will begin to understand why we are just beginning to imagine, from a scientific perspective, how causing stress to the liver can contribute to skin disorders and inflammation (*see Illustration page 75*).

How the Liver Works

Think of the liver as a giant filter for your digestive system. Venous blood that has just picked up digested food from the circulation around the intestines flows first through the liver before entering the general circulation. Kupfer cells, which line the inside of the blood vessels within the liver, actively take up particles and chemicals that need to be removed. Those are then passed into the cells of the body of the liver (parenchyma), where they are prepared for export from the body.

This is done by a chemical modification process to either make them more soluble in water for removal via the kidneys, or to have a "reactive" handle to which a carrier molecule can attach to "lug" them out of the body in the stool.

Since there are many different chemicals, drugs, toxins, and allergens that the liver has to process, there are also many different "chemical machines" to do the job of what is known as "phase I" liver activity. Toxic chemicals that are oil-soluble are made water-soluble by oxidation or by other chemical transformations in phase I liver detoxification. What are the chemicals that we need to get rid of? Think of the Pollutants as the Ps: petrochemicals, pharmaceuticals, PCBs, phenobarbital, pesticides, and poisons from outgassing of furniture and carpets. Chemicals that are otherwise hard to remove have a chemical coupler added by the p450 "mixed-function oxidase" system in phase I.

These phase I p450 enzymes can be activated by certain drugs, herbs, and chemicals in food. Their action also can be slowed by chemicals in ordinary food, resulting in slower breakdown and thus higher levels of certain drugs in the body when those foods are eaten. This is the reason for the warnings about eating grapefruit with certain drugs, which are broken down by the p450 enzyme known as 3A4. A whole class of drugs reaches higher levels in the blood if taken when eating grapefruit, which slows down the action of p450 3A4 enzyme. These include protease inhibitors, antibiotics related to erythromycin, azole antifungals, cancer chemotherapy drugs, benzodiazepines used for anxiety, statin drugs, SSRIs, and many more. Eating grapefruit can make them toxic to people who are more sensitive to elevated levels of these drugs. Eating grapefruit with such medications also has been a risky method attempted by some people in an effort to reduce the dosages of drugs as a cost-saving measure. I use the term risky because it is hard to know what dose of drug and grapefruit to use to have proper effect without toxicity.

To complicate the effects of foods such as grapefruit even further, active compounds have been found that affect two other more recently discovered biochemical systems. P-glycoprotein is involved in the transport of molecules across the cell membranes in organs such as the liver and intestines. Organic ion transporting polypeptides (OATPs) also play a role. Some foods such as grapefruit affect the levels of drugs in the body by influencing not only the p450 enzymes, but by influencing the P-glycoproteins and OATPs to magnify the changes in the same direction.

Other drugs, such as phenobarbital and alcohol, and food substances such as the burnt edges of barbecued meat, push p450 enzymes into high gear, causing more rapid phase I metabolism (breakdown) and activation of whole classes of different compounds. If the more reactive toxins produced by excessive phase I action are not coupled with phase II compounds (see next paragraph), they can react with other chemicals in the body and cause damage. I hope this gives you a tiny taste of how what you eat and are exposed to can affect the activity of drugs and chemicals in your body. In an article I wrote in *Clinics in Dermatology*, I discussed how "naringenin" from grapefruit slowed p450 3A4 and how nobiletin from oranges sped it up, concluding that how you mixed your fruit salad had a lot to do with how you would metabolize a whole classes of drugs. More recent animal data suggests that nobiletin from oranges does not slow down p450 metabolism of compounds, but does not speed it up either.

Phase I liver metabolism, making compounds more reactive, is very helpful if phase II, the combining with a carrier molecule, takes place properly. Think of the carrier molecule as a sort of chemical "locomotive" that couples onto a freight car to tug it away. There are a number of different types of chemical locomotives. These include amino acids, such as glutathione and other sulfur compounds, and glucuronic acid. When these are available, they combine and tug their "freight" into the stool or to the kidneys. When they are scarce, those chemicals and toxins, made even more able to combine with body chemicals, may enter the circulation and attach in places where they wreak havoc. This is just one reason some individuals who start the wrong program for their liver or detox begin to experience worsening of symptoms in what may be labeled a detox reaction. This was seen with some of the first supplemental foods designed to enhance p450 metabolism. Unfortunately, they did not enhance phase II sufficiently. UltraClear by Metagenics, for instance, caused headaches and other reactions in some already toxic people, resulting in the creation of UltraClear Plus, which supplied an excess of chemical locomotives and other factors to favor phase II liver export, eliminating that side effect.

There are a number of supplements that are sold to enhance phase II. There are also a number of supplements, such as MSM, which serve as sulfur sources and may in part be effective because they work in the body as the raw materials needed to make the locomotives for phase II. Sulfur-containing vegetables in the onion family and cabbage family are valuable for phase II clearing. The need for these compounds in the diet is one reason various "detox" products and foods have replaced fasting as the most efficient way to clear out unwanted chemicals and toxins. There are also herbs and foods which speed up phase II liver detox, such as watercress and artichoke. Silymarin (milk thistle), one of the best liver herbs, has been shown in scientific studies to slow down P450 3A4.

Be aware that a number of drugs inhibit p450 enzymes, including common ones such as erythromycin, sulfonamides, fluconazole, and metronidazole. Other drugs induce these enzymes and make them work faster. Alcohol can have one effect or another, depending on how it is used. Binge drinking can inhibit p450 enzymes, while chronic alcohol use can induce them. There are many people today who have liver damage resulting from excessive use of alcohol and even from excessive sugar consumption.

There is another complication that arises from the liver metabolizing and eliminating these various substances: all this activity generates free radicals. If you have sufficient antioxidants available—especially antioxidants such as silymarin that gravitate to the liver—you will have no problem handling the free radical production. But if you are someone whose illness pattern has already thrown you into oxidative stress and you lack the liver-specific antioxidants, you may end up with a detox reaction.

If you are getting the picture that foods are more than just fuel, building blocks, and replacement of missing substances, but are regulators of how our body works and what genes are tuning on in our liver and other organs, you are beginning to see the actual complexity of the effects of our diet on our skin and body.

Illustration
The Liver is Both a Filter and a Processing Facility

What does the liver do? Your blood flows through the digestive tract, moving through the liver before returning to the heart (where it is then pumped through the rest of the body). Your liver filters the blood and removes chemicals, toxins, microbes, and other materials from the blood. The liver acts like a factory to process the toxins that have been removed; it prepares them for "export" by chemically altering them so that they can be coupled to carrier molecules. After they are attached to carrier molecules the liver expels them from the body, by way of the kidneys, the bile, or the stool.

Liver is both filter and processing factory

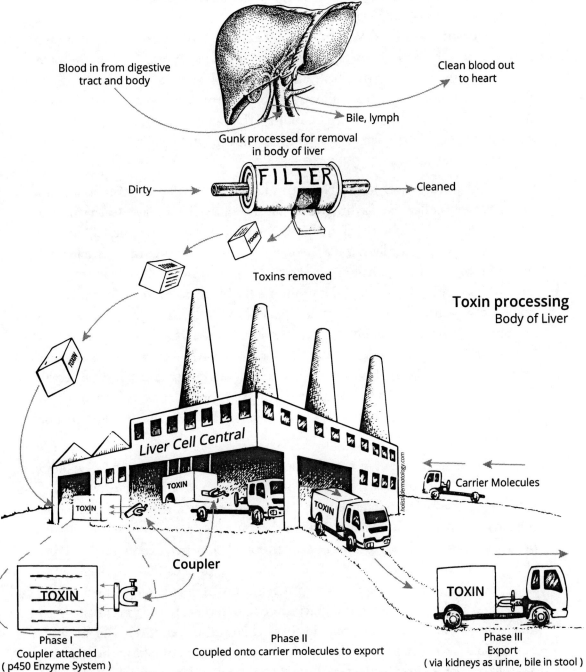

Blood in from digestive tract and body

Clean blood out to heart

Bile, lymph

Gunk processed for removal in body of liver

FILTER

Dirty

Cleaned

Toxins removed

Toxin processing
Body of Liver

Liver Cell Central

holistidermatology.com

TOXIN

Carrier Molecules

Coupler

TOXIN

Phase I
Coupler attached
(p450 Enzyme System)

Phase II
Coupled onto carrier molecules to export

Phase III
Export
(via kidneys as urine, bile in stool)

Fat toxins must be made soluble to be excreted, so they are oxidized to become water soluble. Thus a chemical "coupler" must be added (Phase I) to these toxins, so that they can attach to a carrier molecule (Phase II) and be removed from the body (Phase III).

© Alan M Dattner, MD 2015

75

What to Take

The cautions I have outlined are most important when you are taking pharmaceuticals that have a specific range of action and toxicity. For example, if its breakdown is slowed down too much, an anti-coagulant might thin your blood to the point of bleeding. If you are taking herbs along with certain medications, they must be used very cautiously. If you are on immunosuppressants, for example, some herbs may increase the medication's metabolic breakdown and cause the body to reject a transplanted kidney. St. John's Wort can cause some antiviral AIDS medications to break down too rapidly, changing their effectiveness. Do not begin taking herbal supplements unless you know how they may react with your important medications.

The gentlest liver herb I use is dandelion root. It can be taken as a drink with a vaguely coffee-like flavor (roasted, as in Dandy-Blend), as a tea, a tincture, or a capsule. As mentioned earlier, silymarin is probably one of the best all-around herbs for supporting the liver. It is a flavonoid, so it quenches free radicals generated by the biochemical process of exporting substances from the liver. It protects the liver against toxic substances, and it promotes the biochemical steps for the regeneration of a damaged liver. In short, it is beneficial for the liver alone or in combination with other liver-supportive herbs. And it is used as a food, and has rarely been reported to cause side effects. Turmeric, regularly used in preparation of curry, is another food that is rich in anti-oxidant activity that has liver protective effects. Many herbs traditionally classified as "blood cleansers," such as the Ayurvedic herb Manjista, have been shown in scientific studies to enhance function of the liver.

An early treatment to take the load off the liver was fasting (no new foods to deal with or leak across the gut wall does take some pressure off the liver). Since the body uses stored fat to burn during fasting, fat-soluble toxins such as pesticides, solvents, and petrochemicals dissolved in that fat get released into the circulation during the process. The problem is, as mentioned elsewhere, getting rid of these and other toxic substances in the body is an active process that requires fuel to carry the toxins out; antioxidants to protect against the free radicals generated; and amino acids, glutathione, and glucuronic acid to pull out the bio-transformed toxins. In fasting, you do not take in these chemical locomotives, and the liver cannot do its job of cleaning house efficiently. You also do not take in the anti-oxidants to protect the liver while it generates free radicals during its work of preparing chemicals for export. Besides the Metagenics UltraClear products mentioned above, any number of supplement companies have since created detox products that contain antioxidants, minerals, amino acids, and other phase II locomotives and liver and bile support, and are all helpful in removal of toxic substances from the body.

Another technique I occasionally use to help the liver in people who have had lots of exposure to oil-soluble toxins is the use of castor oil packs. Wool flannel or a similar cloth is soaked in castor oil and placed over the liver on the right upper abdomen. A plastic sheet is placed over the cloth, and a hot water bottle or heating pad is then put on top of the area for an hour or so. This favors chemicals and solvents in the liver and surrounding fat migrating from the liver and into the oil pack. It is best done two to three times a week, especially after other treatments designed to pull toxic fat-soluble substances away from the tissues to which they are bound. One fairly toxic patient I treated with a high dose detox tea blew up with a ¾ inch swelling under his armpit right afterward. I had him follow his use of the detox tea with castor oil packs to remove the toxic chemicals he freed up from where they were bound in his tissues, and prevent further events of that sort. Think of it this way: you can't just ask a badly-behaved partygoer to leave; you must usher him out the door as well. So too, with substances removed by the liver—you must usher them all the way out of the body.

One patient I used this on had spent his entire work life spraying paint in a paint spray booth. He told me that the flannel cloth he put over his liver actually changed color after he did his first treatment. My deep regret is that he threw it away, and we never got an analysis of the contents of that cloth and the substance that dissolved in the castor oil.

The liver flush is a more intense, time consuming, challenging, and occasionally risky method of removing material from the gall bladder and liver. This involves a number of steps that need to be done in proper sequence to avoid obstructing the bile duct with a bile stone pushed out by the flush. The process results in collection of green translucent balls in the stool. Although these are probably not gallstones as touted in descriptions of the process, doctors who I know claim to have seen reduction in the size of the gall bladder (as seen on ultrasound) following the procedure. I have done this with one patient who was also an old friend, who was trying to avoid recommended gall bladder surgery. I knew that there was a small risk of obstruction, but was comforted knowing that she already had an informed surgeon on call to do the surgery in case she plugged her bile duct with a stone. You should be sure to cover your risks if you do a liver flush.

Which Skin Diseases Need Help for the Liver

The real question should be which people need help for the liver. People who have had or currently have their liver compromised by some form of hepatitis are much more likely to need extra support for their liver. Hepatitis can be caused by infections or toxic chemicals. Viral hepatitis has been divided into different types with different modes of transmission. Hepatitis A is caused by oral-fecal contact, and occurs from really poor hygiene, eating raw shellfish from contaminated waters, and unsanitary food workers. Hepatitis B is caused by contact with contaminated blood from transfusions, IV drug use, and contaminated needle sticks. Hepatitis C is usually associated with IV drug use, and sharing of needles, even just once. Blood tests will show antibodies to the type of virus involved, the presence of viral particles, and changes in liver function tests that reflect actual breakdown of the liver. These liver enzyme tests are elevated during, and to a lesser extent, after, the actual illness. The yellow color that often occurs in the skin and eyes of people with hepatitis is caused by elevated levels of bilirubin (from bile) in the blood, which can be seen on blood tests as well.

People who have been exposed to toxic substances as part of their work, home, or hobbies are suspected to have liver damage if skin problems arose after those exposures accumulated. This is truer if they are "sensitive," indicating that they have more trouble breaking down the toxic substances present in our environment. These could include paint fumes, pesticides, animal dander, a moldy house, a toxic work environment, and so forth.

Physicians are so used to patients with obvious liver damage that they overlook patients with compromises in liver function that do not show up via the usual suspects: elevations of liver enzymes in the blood, enlarged liver on x-ray, or by feeling the belly. These changes involve the inability to breakdown inflammatory and toxic substances at the usual rate of speed, so that these substances can accumulate in the body and cause harm. When I first studied medicine, tests were still being performed that were developed before the modern liver enzyme tests. Those tests measured the *function* of the liver in breaking down a chemical called Brom-sulphthalein (BSP).

One of the tests done by functional medical laboratories for the evaluation of the liver involves the measurement of the rate of breakdown of caffeine and acetaminophen by the liver. Despite the history of this concept and its proof in more recent testing, the idea of reduced liver function with otherwise normal enzymes is still not understood by most physicians and patients. It is this gap in understanding/belief that is treated by those who practice beyond the realm of conventional medicine. But the common sense understanding of this concept and the scientific basis of it is there to be discovered by anyone who searches.

Anyone with contributory digestive issues, who for years has a "leaky gut" (described in Chapter 6) with foreign "antigens" leaking into the circulation, will certainly have overwhelmed their liver. Because of that, I find that some kind of support for the liver is a foundational part of my correcting skin and inflammatory diseases in anyone who has had chronic leaky gut or food sensitivity issues.

Tom's Story

When I first started practice at a clinic run by the Integral Yoga Center, a boy I'll call Tom came in with a strange rash with lesions in different stages of development, including crusted areas where the tiny blood vessels in the skin had broken down. From my recent training, I recognized this rash to be a specific condition with a name which was one of the biggest mouthfuls to pronounce that we had ever learned as budding dermatologists: *pityriasis lichenoides et variolformis acuta*, or PLEVA. No one knew the cause of the condition. Various treatments sometimes worked, or the condition went away on its own. Dr. Sandy McClanahan, the head physician of the clinic, came in, muscle-tested the patient, and recommended a series of supplements, one of which was for treatment of the liver. To the surprise of all of us, Tom improved rapidly over the next two weeks and his condition cleared. I presented him at grand Rounds at Brown University, and the dermatologists there were fascinated and took notes on the substances used to treat the liver and other organs in this condition. However, as I found out when I was fated to get my next patient with this unusual condition, the defects and needed remedies were specific to the patient and not to the disease. The next boy with PLEVA did not respond to the same supplements.

The same liver and other organ treatment regimen that brought a rapid resolution in one patient with this disease did not give any visible results in the next. The importance of helping the liver may vary from individual to individual with the same "disease" but it is important to treat when its sluggishness is contributing to the condition at hand.

The Liver and the Skin

If the information presented so far does not convince you that there is a relationship between the liver and the skin, you may be surprised to learn that scientific studies have demonstrated that most of the p450 enzymes are found in human skin tissue; the skin was obtained either by biopsy or in examination of cultures of component skin cells such as keratinocytes, fibroblasts, or melanocytes. This information helps close the loop on the notion that the skin helps take over when the liver is overwhelmed, and that skin disease may be an expression of that overwhelmed status. The skin does not have the same level of capability of biotransforming toxins that the liver does, so it is not exactly a second liver. But the presence of p450 enzymes in skin indicates that it can form more reactive compounds from the toxins it is trying to get rid of, and these may be responsible for some of the rashes we see.

As you improve the function of the liver you will change how everything is broken down. Clearly, you will affect the potency of any pharmaceutical drugs in your system. You may get more toxic if your phase II elimination does not keep up with your p450 conjugation of substances, or if the generation of free radicals by enhanced liver metabolism overwhelms your previous capacity to "quench" or dampen the level of free radicals through antioxidants in your system.

For some people, initiating change, getting the liver working better, and getting bound toxins released is like stirring up a hornet's nest. You have to usher the hornets out to prevent getting stung. Complete removal of toxic molecules from inside the body, a function of the liver, requires proper activity of the bowels, kidneys, and bile system to complete the process. Making sure that there is no constipation, and that the other organs are functioning well is crucial. Some people grease the pathways for release best by using homeopathic drainage remedies for the different organs involved. Consider this if you get "toxic" when first taking herbs that support the liver.

Summary

If you are getting the idea that the function of the liver is complex, you are reading correctly. Many physicians do not understand the basics of Phase I and Phase II liver detoxification. Predicting actual effects of multiple drugs on the metabolism of other drugs can be a daunting task, even when you are knowledgeable and have support of studies in the medical literature.

Nevertheless, there are some principles you should understand from this chapter if you are to seek natural treatment of skin disease or inflammation in the body. First, with the 80,000 legal chemicals in our environment, food, air, and water, the liver is expected to be under stress and need support. Leaking of incompletely digested foods across the intestinal barrier into the blood flowing to the liver aggravates this situation further, and requires liver support to successfully remedy the problem. Second, fasting may take the food-derived load off the liver, but also may remove needed food-derived support. The right detox food can help with this process, as long as there are not allergens or sensitizers in the products. Third, supporting phase II with the right chemical "locomotives" to tug out activated toxins can be very important in turning off skin disorders, inflammatory reactions, and all sorts of unexplained symptoms. Finally, when someone's health is dependent on the exact concentrations of one or more drugs they are taking, herbs, supplements, and even big changes in diet must be added with caution because of the possibility that they could cause the liver to alter the concentration of those crucial drugs in the body. My medical training taught me how to evaluate the liver, but I had to study herbs and functional medicine to learn how to treat it. We now have many options for helping an over-stressed liver regain normal function, and help the skin function better as a result. This chapter is an introduction to those options.

Part 2

SKIN AND SKIN CONDITIONS

CHAPTER 7
THE SKIN AS A REFLECTION OF THE WHOLE BEING

How your skin looks is a direct reflection of how well your body is functioning. Nearly every rash is a reflection of some process gone awry internally. Your skin provides back-up support to the kidneys, liver, lungs, and intestine, helping getting rid of unwanted substances. When these organs are not functioning properly, the burden may be placed on skin. Oxidative stress, vascular weakness, hormonal imbalances, autoimmune conditions, allergy, and metabolic imbalances all show up in the skin. So does unresolved stress, through a variety of pathways, from digestive weakness to adrenal fatigue to muscular exhaustion. They can all contribute to the skin and face looking and feeling worn out. The skin is very much like the dashboard of your car, flashing the red "check engine" light when there are problems under the hood. This book gives you information on how to read those warning lights, and what to do about them.

The Skin as a Reflection of Your Inner Workings

A classical textbook on dermatology, Dr. Irwin Braverman's *Skin Signs of Systemic Diseases,* looks at skin conditions as the body telling us that something is wrong inside. This text is a compilation of both common and rare disorders that can be detected by various signs and conditions on the skin. For example, there are conditions such as Ehlers-Danlos syndrome where super-stretchy skin on the elbows, resulting from defects in the elastic tissue formation, serves as a warning that blood vessels inside the body may have defects and be more likely to burst than usual. Many other internal conditions involving genetic and subsequent biochemical, cell, and organ defects can be spotted because of telltale findings on the skin.

Various signs on the fingernails, skin, and hair are sometimes associated with particular conditions. The alternative medical world is full of these signs. For example, pale or whitish spots on fingernails were supposed to be a sign of zinc deficiency. However, although this may be true in some cases, white spots can also be an indication of injury or other causes. As a result of the variety of causes for a given condition, many signs on the skin may best be used to pose a specific question rather than to provide an answer.

Different healing systems also provide formulas for interpreting findings on the skin. For example, Chinese and Ayurvedic medicine both offer methods to interpret the shape, color, grooves and appearance of the tongue as a reflection of what is going on in the digestive system and elsewhere. Appearance of the skin, and various patterns seen, such as fingerprints, palm lines, earlobe creases and many more have been interpreted by different schools as having predictive ability to the state of the individual.

Some skin signs are well accepted quite universally, and are ones you are likely aware of. Jaundice, or yellow color of the skin, will tell you of liver disease. Yellow palms may be a sign of eating too many carrots.

Skin Conditions as a Sign of Something Awry Inside

One foundational principle on which this book is based is that improper handling of allergic and toxic substances leads to inflammation of the skin. The skin acts as a backup for other organs of elimination such as the bowel, kidneys, liver, and lungs, and when these organs are overloaded or not functioning well, the skin takes over eliminating toxins, and sometimes erupts at the task. Furthermore, since food entering the digestive system is the largest source of foreign material entering the body, it is vital to correct both the foods taken in and the activity of the gut in processing them, to remove the stimuli for inflammatory skin conditions. I can't support the idea that inflammation just "happens" without any knowable reason and can only be controlled by suppression of the immune response.

Most of the specific details about how the skin reflects problems in your digestive system, liver, kidneys, immune system, and psychological/emotional/spiritual dynamics, are discussed in other chapters.

Skin: The Boundary Between Self and Other

Your skin is the key junction and boundary between self and not self. This includes the metaphorical as well as the physical. Exploring our collective metaphors about skin can help us understand unconscious ways we think about and treat our skin. We say that people who have become immune to rejection are "thick-skinned." When we want to remind ourselves about the importance of a good personality, we say beauty is only "skin-deep." When a person causes us to feel annoyance or affection, we say "they've gotten under my skin."

Skin is a moving boundary as well. After a sunburn, people often see a layer of dead skin peel off. Let's look at the skin from the eyes of the reptile: when someone grows beyond old limitations, they are like a snake shedding its old skin. And now, consider the skin from the viewpoint of a dust mite that lives off particles of skin. The skin is in a constant process of renewing itself. We can be likened to biologic ambassadors. Wherever we go, we literally leave part of ourselves as the surface skin cells die and slough off.

As a cultural boundary, the color of one's skin has enabled slavery, racism, and discrimination. For thousands of years, people have tattooed and pierced the skin to send cultural, political, emotional, and spiritual messages to the world, or to mark important touchstones or events in life. The nine pounds of skin and nerves on the body's surface occupy a significant space in the brain where we feel pleasure, pain, pressure, itching, and other subtle sensations that make up the landscape of our perception of being touched.

The health of the skin, not just its appearance, is an important metaphor for the health of one's boundary between self and other. Truly healthy skin acts as a membrane that lets appropriate molecules in and keeps inappropriate molecules out, on all levels. When you meet a person, the first thing you see is their skin. It may envelop familiar structures that you recognize, but you are actually looking at the person's skin and not those structures. Just as clothing wraps the skin, the skin wraps those underlying structures, whether the person is a "bag of bones" or a muscular weight lifter.

You see a lot of things besides the overall shape of the skin. You see changes of texture from old scars, from acne, or from too much time in the sun. You see lines from repeated expressions of emotions in the past, and lines from particular emotions the person is experiencing in real time as you interact with them. Changes in skin color can reveal emotions: people get red with embarrassment, green with disgust, or white with fear. Colors reflect their vitality or illness. The pasty pale individual looks very different from the same individual well and full of vitality. The smell of the skin, too, upon release of hormones, can communicate anxiety, arousal, and other biological and emotional messages.

There are many subtle levels on which information is communicated, and they may be telegraphed beyond the visual appearance of the skin. Clearly, more information is conveyed by the skin than just its shape and surface pattern at a given time. In fact, you see so many things as you look at an individual's skin, including all the changes and expressions it goes through, that you may integrate information from that viewing which is more than the sum total of all of the signals you can recall. In one "blink," you get a powerful impression of that individual.

How else is the skin a pivotal aspect of your anatomy? Although mentioning the skin as the "largest organ" usually brings out some nervous giggles from a class of early teenagers, it actually is the largest organ, because it has so much to cover and so many functions to perform in that process. Here I will remind you of some of those functions that you almost instinctively know, and fill in some details of how the skin accomplishes them. The more you understand about the skin, the better equipped you will be to make choices for your own health.

Where Exactly Do "You" Begin?

Our "self" does not completely stop at the brick and mortar layer of the epidermis. In many different ways, part of us extends out beyond that border, much as the headlights coming out from a car. The headlights might correspond to the subtle electromagnetic energy field that emanates from our electrochemical makeup, or to our emotional nature, which attracts and repels others. We emit chemicals as odors, we breathe in and out, and studies show bacteria and other microbes not only live in our skin, but also surround our bodies in a kind of haze. We talk of people getting into our space, or getting into our face, when they get too close. And we stay away from infected people because of what they cough and breathe out, and what is on their skin. Some people concretize this outer layer into an "aura," and there are some people who claim to be able to see and describe the auras around other people.

Still, the most agreed-upon location where "outside" or "other" stops and "you" begins is the outer layer of the skin. As an interface, the skin is a kind of focal point between the world outside of you and the world inside you; it defines where space starts being you.

Deep Knowing Emanates from Beneath the Skin

I want to break from my discussion here to discuss the nature of the process of deep knowing from which action comes. Understanding that cigarettes cause cancer is something a lot of smokers *know* but dismiss for various reasons. They don't stop because they do not *know it* in the deepest sense. I knew that driving too fast for icy conditions was dangerous, but despite a few skids and spin-outs, I did not know it deep enough. That was until my tires broke loose from the road during a snow storm, and I hit a tree sideways and wound up squished with a lot of broken parts and pain. Today I *know* the dangers of snowy roads in the deepest part of my being, and have driven much more slowly and more cautiously for the past 28 winters.

Years in the laboratory also taught me a lot. But it took nearly three years at NIH, watching evidence pour out of our data demonstrating the nature and reality of lymphocytic cross-reactive recognition for me to *know* in the depth of my being that this was the reality of how our cellular immune system works. Finally, I understood this process really occurs and is the cause of much of the allergy and inflammation we see in the skin and other disorders. Again, here, I really knew in the deepest sense, and have felt compelled to apply this reality in looking for the specific causes of an individual's inflammation ever since. Many of my colleagues have seen publications on this subject in the past few years, but since it is not deeply embedded in them as a truth, they do not seek or act on this information in seeking the cause of inflammatory conditions in the process of treating patients.

The Skin as Barrier

The skin is a major barrier between you and the environment on a number of different levels. That skin is the absolute beginning of you. On any part of your body that is not covered by clothing, the sunlight reflects off your skin. So does the moonlight, the twilight and the kitchen light. Skin is a barrier, an absorber, and a reflector of light. Your skin prepares activated vitamin D from light, and prepares melanin to darken itself and prevent the entry of excessive light.

Your skin is a barrier for light, as well. When you look at yourself in the mirror after a shower, you see the light reflected off the surface of your skin. When you see the faces of others, you are looking first at their skin. It is the subtle colors of the skin, and the emotions expressed through the facial expressions and changes in blood flow, that give the impression of being radiant.

This barrier protects you from invading bacteria and other microorganisms. It prevents the loss of water and bodily fluids such as lymph and blood. It seals up and heals over when there are cuts and abrasions. It signals the immune system components when there are threats from chemicals and microorganisms. It also protects you from certain forms of radiation, such as ultraviolet light.

Viewing skin conditions as a means for the body to tell us that something is wrong inside may sound simplistic to physicians and dermatologists, but there has been a growing body of knowledge that supports this hypothesis. It has been supported in specific instances, in the past, by Dr. Braverman's text, *Skin Signs of Systemic Disease*, and additional related reports in the literature. Advancement of understanding of how the body works at a molecular level has demonstrated that the skin performs many of the same chemical processes as other organs in the body. I find it fascinating that deeper scientific understanding of the skin and underlying organs brings us closer to understanding that skin conditions are related to malfunction of those organs.

From an entirely different direction, herbalists have looked at the skin as excreting toxic substances that have overwhelmed the internal organs. They look at the skin as an accessory organ of excretion, with skin conditions arising because the skin is getting rid of toxins that the organs of removal in the body cannot handle. As a remedy for this problem, they use herbs that increase the function of the organs of excretion, such as the kidney and liver.

Modern science has shown that the sweat ducts in the skin do operate very similarly to the tubules in the kidney. The kidneys are the structures that filter the blood and remove wastes such as urea and excess sodium and other minerals. The tubules in which this process occurs are complex structures that first excrete waste substances into the tube for removal, and in the last portion of the tubule, reabsorb into the body those minerals and chemicals which the body wants to retain. It has to be more than a coincidence that the sweat ducts operate in exactly the same way. Wastes are excreted into the sweat duct in the proximal (closer in) portion, and then nutrients are reabsorbed from the duct in the distal (further out) portion before the sweat is deposited on the skin.

Sounds pretty similar, doesn't it? Also, there are about as many sweat glands in one's skin as there are tubules in one kidney. Purists would argue that the actions in the tubules in the kidney are controlled by hormones, which do not influence the sweat ducts. Either way, it's easy to consider that the sweat ducts are excreting materials that have overwhelmed the kidney's capacity, and that if they are toxic or allergenic, those materials sit on the skin and cause trouble.

The skin also has amazing similarities to the rest of the body with regard to response to hormones and other chemical signals, and also in the production and regulation of many of these signals. For example, production of vitamin D and regulation of the production of steroids are among the hormone functions that make the skin the largest external endocrine organ. Cholesterol synthesis and regulation of its conversion into sex hormones also takes place in sebaceous glands of the skin. These are just a few examples of the many ways in which the skin participates in the production and modification of signal systems in the body.

Summary

As you can see from this chapter, there are numerous ways in which both genetic and environmental conditions are reflected in the skin. The skin acts as a barrier, controlling the transfer of light, heat, water, chemicals, and microbes across it into the body. It has its own population of microbes, influencing the microbes and immune system of the body. It acts as a third kidney, in eliminating unwanted substances from the skin. And it participates in the production and regulation of hormones and numerous chemical signals throughout the body. It can no longer be viewed as just a protective coating, but rather it must be viewed as both a mirror of internal body processes and as an active crucial participant in the control of function of the body.

CHAPTER 8

CULTIVATING BEAUTY, OUTSIDE AND IN

We often forget that our skin is an amazing reflector of our whole selves—body and soul. The kind of life a person has led frequently shows up in his or her face; we don't need to know personal details to know if someone's been through difficult times or had a rough life. Problems in our lives often lay the groundwork for problems with our skin.

Of course, not all of our wrinkles and skin conditions come from lifestyle choices or circumstances. Many of our problems begin with the nutritional choices we make. Have you ever noticed that problem foods "bite back"? Take, for example, that high-sugar chewy candy you know is bad for you. It inevitably gets stuck in a bad tooth and leaves it aching for days. And what about that carbonated sugar-laden beverage that picks you up for fifteen minutes, then drops you like a sack of potatoes so that you can't get out of your chair? Personally, eating a full portion of fried food gives me a certain kind of heaviness in the head, discomfort in the gut, and an overall feeling of lethargy. Think of how you react to fried or other problem foods and you'll quickly see how the choices you make have palpable, and often visible, consequences.

Some conditions caused by old eating habits can be cleared up with the proper medication. For instance, you can use steroid creams for a rash or antibiotics for your acne. They may clear up the condition, but it often comes back after you stop the drug. And if you have not gotten to the root of the problem, it will grow as does a weed in a summer garden whose roots grow deeper as it comes back again and again. The drugs may work when your ability to let go of harmful habits does not, but you will eventually suffer the consequences of both the bad habit and the drug. Soon, you will have a new set of problems to solve. These build in layers, and have to be unwound strand by strand to restore some sort of normal balance.

Not everyone can get back to that balance. Some people have suffered too much damage, and can only do their best to make partial changes. If you are not too far gone, and you feel that your life is worth it, consider taking the best steps forward that you can. No one is perfect, so you will have to honestly observe how far you can stray from a healing program without a massive setback.

Nutrition and Aging

Perhaps one of the topics that garners me the most phone calls from magazine writers is the subject of what to eat to slow aging and stay young and beautiful looking. To understand the answer to this question, it is necessary to consider some of the changes that take place in your skin as you age. I will discuss a number of reasons that skin develops an aged appearance, but first I will describe some of the changes that occur on biochemical, physiologic, and inflammatory levels. In other words, I am going to give you a scientific explanation of aging so that you can better make choices to slow the process and evaluate the claims of diverse potions that will undoubtedly be offered to you at various times during your life.

Let us zoom in on the changes in aging skin as if we are moving down to earth from outer space, looking at the different levels of structure as we get closer.

From afar, loss of the framework made up of bone structure, muscle, and subcutaneous fat of the face can cause an appearance of sagging of the inner cheeks and mouth. Getting closer, we see large wrinkles that result from the repeated action of the muscles of expression. As both collagen and elastin (the material that helps young skin spring back to its original shape after stretching) are lost, fine wrinkles appear around the eyes. We will zoom in and take a closer look at this important process as we get closer to the biochemical structure of the skin. Thinning of the skin and dryness occurs in the elderly, as both the cells of the outermost layer of the skin (the epidermis) and the tough inner layer (the dermis) become weakened and fatigued, and lose their vigor.

Let's return to the sagging, and the elastic tissue that prevents sagging. You probably have had the experience of having a bathing suit or underwear with built-in elastic waistband. As you pull the garment on, the elastic stretches to fit your body; when you take it off, the elastic snaps back to its original shape. After a few years of washing and wearing, something happens to that elastic material, and the waistband stretches out and no longer returns to its shape. That is a somewhat similar to what happens in your skin when its "elastic fibers" fail to work properly.

Loss of elasticity happens not only from breakdown of the elastic material, but also from the loss of the attachments and the suspension network that gave it the stretchiness in the first place. Imagine a cot with all the springs attached around the edge of the wire center. It gives good stretchy support, but the longer you have the cot, the fewer functional springs remain, until the cot is no longer suspended or stretchy. Our skin, which, "out of the factory," has elastic fibers just as does the cot, is suspended in two dimensions—but it also has fine elastic fibers that anchor it to deep structures in a third dimension. It is the loss of all of these fibers that leads to diminished elasticity and fine wrinkling.

Biochemistry of Skin Aging: Free Radicals and Oxidation

Let's examine still deeper layers to see what is happening on the chemical level for such changes to occur. For this we have to look at what scientists have discovered about the process.

Part of the thick layer of the skin, or dermis, is made up of elastic tissue fibers that function like a rubber support skeleton around the skin structures to help return the skin to its original shape after stretching. Collagen fibers give the skin the remainder of its strength. Aging, and more specifically, chemical damage known as **oxidation** and **free radical** damage leads to a series of events that cause the fragmentation of these elastic tissue fibers.

Free radicals are molecules that have an uneven number of electrons, so they are always *searching* for an extra electron they can "steal" to become stable. They start a chain reaction, turning molecules they bump against into more free radicals. This process keeps repeating itself until lots of chemical structures have been made into reactive free radicals. The chemical structures that become free radicals combine with each other (cross-link) and with molecules in the structure of your skin in ways that shouldn't occur except in advanced aging.

Before we continue, let me just state that it must be a product of their desire to appear more human and retain their sense of humor that has caused scientists to choose the names they have for these chemicals of aging. You see, one path to aging involves the alteration of our tissues via the attachment of particular chemicals. These combination age-related chemicals are called Advanced Glycation

End products or "AGEs" in scientific jargon. They serve as a key in a lock for certain other chemical machines known as enzymes, which, when started on their rampage, chew up the elastin or collagen. The receptors for these AGEs are known as Receptors for Advanced Glycation End products, or RAGES. I can just imagine the smiles on researchers' faces as they publish some very "dry" scientific studies on the emotionally-charged topic of aging with AGE-RAGE in the title.

As I said, the "G" in AGEs stands for glycation, the process by which sugar "gloms onto" or binds to protein, which happens when sugar levels are too high. A series of chemical reactions eventually form the AGEs that trigger the enzymes to chomp up the elastin and collagen, leaving a saggy mess.

A lot of research on this topic comes from the study of diabetes; however, it turns out that sugar is not the only substance that can form AGEs. Heating fat and protein to high temperature, as in frying, can do the same. It has also been shown that we absorb AGEs from the food we eat. In other words, not only do dangerous food components we eat (such as extra sugar) attach to the chemicals of our body and transform them, but we absorb attached chemicals that are already in the food we eat, creating later problems including attacks by our immune system, which does not recognize our changed body chemicals.

AGEs send signals to enzymes in our skin to break down the structural collagen (which gives skin its strength) and elastin (which allows the skin to spring back to its original shape). These enzymes, known as "metalloproteases" (molecular shredders in the tissue), chomp up the collagen and elastic tissue and cause the disintegration of the elastic nature of the skin, leading to thinning, wrinkling, and sagging. This is a vicious process, activated by sunlight and accelerated by damage from unhealthy foods and other oxidative stresses such as smoking. Inflammation can also activate these metalloproteases to chomp up collagen and elastic tissue.

Under the microscope, normal elastic tissue in skin appears to be a matrix of woven fibers. Sun damage and aging make it appear broken, clumped, and calcified. Excessive sunshine also leads to production of free radicals and damage to the collagen and elastic tissue as the sun's radiation is absorbed into the skin. As dermatology residents, we learned that we could tell if a stained microscopic skin biopsy was from the face, or another sun-exposed area, by a characteristic bluish color that appeared in the dermis of sun-exposed skin (see chapter 10 for more on sun exposure and sunscreens). So, very real chemical changes take place in the skin from sun damage. Cigarette smoke may also accelerate the skin-aging process because free radicals are present in the burning material. In addition, the fat layer of the skin under the dermis is likely to thin where repetitive creasing occurs. Gravity adds to the sagging caused by thinning of the tissues, and loss of tone of the facial muscles aggravates this.

Another problem related to all of this is the storing of toxic substances. AGEs and other toxic products that do not get excreted have to go somewhere. The body, in its wisdom, does not deposit them in critical-to-life areas such as the brain and heart. Instead, the body binds them to connective tissue (tendons and collagen) in the deep layer of the skin known as the dermis.

Let's add together all these contributions to skin aging at the sub-microscopic level:

- "Foods" such as sugar that bind to the skin and cause AGE formation.

- Sources of AGEs in our diet: sugary treats and crispy fried foods.

- Other toxic substances, such as endotoxins from bacteria, fungal toxins, and toxic chemicals in what we put onto our skin, that have no better place to go.

- Oxidation damage from the sun, food consumption, the process of burning calories, metabolism, the breaking down of toxic chemicals, and inhalation of smog and smoke.

- Emotional distress releasing adrenaline for prolonged amounts of time.

- Physical toxins, such as heavy metals, pesticides, and environmental chemicals, or the effects of chronic fatigue or illness.

- Any source of inflammation of the skin involved

The general reduction of metabolic activity that comes with aging and sun damage slows down the manufacture and repair processes. The effects of inner direction on skin blood flow and metabolism become more apparent as you compare the sallow skin of withdrawn, sick individuals against that of healthy people of the same age.

Prevention

Some of the hottest aspects of skin care are beauty enhancement and the anti-aging measures that are part of creating a vibrant youthful appearance. It has become apparent to me, and I'm sure to you as well, that there are some people in their 60s who look, act, and function similarly to people 15 years younger, and that there are even some people in their 80s who look and function as do people in their 60s (granted, some of this is in their genes). Let's look at some of the measures these "youngsters" take to keep their youthful appearance.

- **Use sunscreen**: One of the most important things you can do to reduce the look of aging skin is to prevent sunburn. You can do this by limiting the length of exposure, by wearing hats, and by using sunscreen. There are now "chemical free" sunscreens on the market that contain little reflective flecks of zinc oxide or titanium oxide. Some evidence suggests that they may be better in the long run than the chemical sunscreens such as PABA esters, oxybenzone, and methyl cinnamates. Sunscreens slow the partial penetration of radiation to allow longer exposure to the sun without burning compared to skin that is unprotected by a sunscreen, which allows you to be out in the sun for a much longer amount of time. Only time will reveal the effectiveness of the sunscreen as the first generation that uses chemical sunscreens becomes aged (see Chapter 10 regarding sun damage and the sunscreen for a more detailed explanation of this issue).

- **Stop smoking**: If you smoke, you will get wrinkles. It's as simple as that. Second-hand smoke may be just as harmful as active smoking in creating crow's feet. Hanging out in smoky bars may be almost as wrinkle-forming as smoking itself.

- **Take appropriate protective supplements**: There are a number of supplements that reduce free radical damage inside the body. The most well-known of these are vitamin C, vitamin E, and mixed carotenoids such as are present in carrots and other orange, yellow, or red fruits and vegetables. Vitamin C in its natural form is often accompanied in plant sources by a number of free radical quenchers known as bioflavonoids. It appears that these free radical quenchers work best all together, or synergistically, rather than each alone, in calming down the excited molecules by passing off the active electron to where it won't do any harm. These supplements also work with free radical quencher chemicals within the human body such as super oxide dismutase (SOD) and reduced glutathione. It is important to mention these other big-name molecules because while it is not clear how well you can absorb SOD when taken by mouth in pill form, it is clear that you can take various building blocks of SOD, such as copper and selenium, as nutritional supplements. Other free radical quenchers and antioxidants include:

  - Proanthocyanidins, an important group of bioflavonoid antioxidants that

RADIANT SKIN: FROM THE INSIDE OUT

occur in the purple skin of grapes, in grape seeds, and in Polypodium leuco-
tomos (a fern from Central America). They protect the fine blood vessels
known as capillaries, as well as the skin.

• Citrus fruits, which contain bioflavonoids of a different sort in their inner
pulp.

• Green tea, which has bioflavonoid antioxidants, the most researched of
which is Epigallocatechin gallate, or EGCG. These have anti-aging and anti-
cancer effects.

• Selenium salts, which are building blocks for antioxidants made in the body.

• N-acetyl-Cysteine (NAC), which is a building block for the important
antioxidant molecule glutathione.

• Lipoic acid, which plays a role in the regeneration of Vitamin C as an
antioxidant.

Although you cannot control all the free radical stresses to which you are
exposed, you can certainly increase your level of antioxidant protection at the
times it is needed. When I take a summer vacation or go south for a week in the
winter, I routinely double or triple the level of antioxidant supplements that I take
on a daily basis, before, during, and after the trip. If my love of music takes me to
a smoky bar, I reduce the negative effect somewhat by afterwards taking extra
vitamin C, antioxidants, and herbs to detoxify my body.

Treatment

Current treatments to enhance beauty certainly yield dramatic improvements in the apparent youthfulness of some people. Unfortunately, not everyone
has good results or is free from the possibility of long-lasting side effects. Surgical
procedures can result in scarring, problems during anesthesia, or interference with
nerves. Lasers can cause damage and pigmentation irregularity. Even Intermittent
Pulsed Light (IPL), which sounds safe enough, has caused fat atrophy in some
patients. Many of the creams sold for moisturizing and anti-aging contain antioxidants and other helpful ingredients. They may also contain preservatives and
emulsifiers and other components that are suspected to be carcinogens or hormone
disrupters (even though they are legal to use). Unfortunately, some beauty models
have found this out when they discovered that they had cancer at an early age.

DIY Non-invasive Treatments

There are certainly less invasive treatments available. Skilled facial massage with the right creams and oils can be very effective in combating the signs of aging. The predominant effect of a facial, beyond the esoteric creams applied, is the relaxation of the muscles of the face and the smoothing of the tension lines and deep creases. I give myself a facial in the shower or hot tub or when washing my face at the sink, massaging facial muscles and letting out whatever groans and sounds of tension that want to emerge. You can experience this massage as a sensual, delicious opportunity to release the tensions of the day you have accumulated in the muscles of your face. Sometimes I do it with progressive deep relaxation, first feeling and then progressively letting go of the tension in my face as I work my way up from my neck, to my mouth to the muscles around my eyes, my brow, and the muscles of my jaw along the sides of my head. Often I am amazed to feel my jaw relax downward and I discover how much tension I had been carrying without even being aware of it.

I once conducted an experiment in my office. For about five days, I rubbed only the left side of my face with a vitamin C preparation followed by vitamin E oil. I was amazed to find that all three members of my staff could identify which side of my face I was treating because of the diminished horizontal lines on that side of my forehead. I believe that in that short a time, the massaging in of the liquids was more important than the composition of the liquids themselves, although these may give further help over the long run.

It's important to remember to enjoy the process rather than think of it as yet another task you have to do.

Topical Applications:

This section is a brief summary of some of the substances that are used in anti-aging products to apply to the skin. It is important to note that many of them also are used orally for that purpose. As you might guess, this is a very large topic on which thousands of articles and books have been written, so it is hard to do justice to the entire topic in one chapter. This section is meant to give you an overview on the scientific thinking and the evolution of that understanding, so that you can understand more about the reality of claims made for various products, and make better choices of what to use to keep your skin looking young.

Most dermatologists do not recommend using oral forms of natural products and herbs; so it is a revelation to find that dermatologists are now recommending a new class of topically applied anti-aging compounds that contains herbs, natural products, and other biological materials (including genetically engineered human growth factors). These are cosmeceuticals—cosmetics that claim to have medicinal (e.g., anti-aging, anti-oxidant, etc.) properties. A major paradox here is that if the anti-aging properties are proven and claimed, the FDA can classify them as drugs, and they can be removed from the market if they have not met the testing required of drugs.

Cosmeceutical Ingredients

It is important to familiarize yourself with the most effective ingredients currently being used and how they work, alone and in combination. This will explain why different products with virtually the same ingredients may have differing levels of effectiveness. In general, ingredients that are really beneficial for the skin should be taken both internally and applied on the surface in the form most appropriate for absorption via the route given. Topical products work well because they are being delivered directly to the site where their activity is desired. The challenge for these products to be most effective is that their chemicals must be delivered through the barrier of the skin and then be released at the level where they can best act.

It is beyond the scope of this chapter to have a full discussion of cosmeceuticals. The following are some of the most widely-used cosmeceutical ingredients:

• **Vitamin A**: Vitamin A products, termed retinoids, have the ability to activate genes to increase the thickness of the skin, as well as "puff out" fine wrinkles by causing a little swelling and thickening of the outer layers. As one of the first products shown to actually restore the thickness of aged skin, retinoids are useful for those who have thinning, aged skin. If one's skin is sensitive, and already red and irritated, topical vitamin A products are not likely to be well tolerated. Since vitamin A topical products cause cells to divide more rapidly, they are not a good choice during the seasons when people are out in the sun, or for people who get a lot of sun exposure, because they can cause abnormal, cancerous cells to divide more rapidly.

- **Antioxidants**: Antioxidant products operate in a variety of ways. Some antioxidants act to activate, or transform genes to start producing their own antioxidants. Some function directly as antioxidants to quench free radicals. Some act as building materials for the body to make its own antioxidants. For example, salts of the mineral selenium, N-acetyl-cysteine, and curcumin (found in turmeric) are building blocks for the body's powerful antioxidant glutathione. And the antioxidant lipoic acid helps in the process of regenerating the capacity of oxidized vitamin C to the form in which it can act as an antioxidant again. Antioxidants benefit skin that is or has been damaged by the sun by the process known as "photo-aging."

- **Vitamin C**: Many anti-aging molecules have a variety of different activities in slowing aging. An example is vitamin C, which is involved directly in calming down free radicals, and is also crucial for the synthesis of elastin and collagen, the substances that give the skin its strength and elasticity. Vitamin C also has anti-inflammatory activity, so it is capable of slowing down some of the inflammatory processes involved in age-related breakdown of the elasticity and structure of the skin. Vitamin C requires an acid pH to penetrate the skin, so formulations that are effective are more acid and can be irritating to some people. There is a delicate balance in formulating an effective product that does not irritate.

It is no accident that vitamin C appears in nature in plants, accompanied by other classes of antioxidants such as "bioflavonoids" (or flavonoids, which are similar to vitamins, are important in maintaining health, in reducing the risk of cancer and heart disease, and in helping the body get rid of toxins). Plants, as can human skin, can be damaged by too much sun, as you may know if you put sprouts or young plants in direct sunlight before they have time to get "conditioned." Conditioning involves gradual exposure to more and more light, and the induction of the production of more green chlorophyll and photo-protective antioxidants, which work in combination with vitamin C to prevent free radical damage. We need this sort of combination of antioxidants in our skin (e.g., vitamin C + bioflavonoids).

An example we learn from history is that the extreme lack of Vitamin C causes scurvy. British sailors learned to counteract this deficiency by eating citrus, which is why they were called "limies." The pulp and white of the lime and other citrus fruits are filled with bioflavonoids, which work along with the vitamin C. French sailors with scurvy along the St. Laurence River in Canada were helped by the Indians, who gave them pine bark to eat, which is rich in a class of bioflavonoids known as oligo proanthocyanidins, or OPCs. Vitamin C and OPCs are both now part of many oral and topical supplements to reduce damage from aging. Related compounds are found in grapes and red wine, and thought to be responsible for the "French Paradox"; that the red-wine-consuming French have a lower level of heart disease than would be expected from the amount of fats they consume when eating.

• **Vitamin B:** B vitamins such as Niacinamide play a role in energy production in skin cells. They also help improve skin surface texture by reducing pore size.

• **Cholesterol:** Another important function of the skin is the formation of a protective barrier to keep the skin from losing water and drying out, and to keep it from absorbing foreign chemicals and bacteria. Free fatty acids, cholesterol, and waxes are synthesized by the skin in the upper layers, to help create this barrier. Ultimately, they are converted to a combination of cholesterol and waxes, known as "ceramides," in the upper layer of the skin. If cholesterol is depleted, the skin cells begin to lose water, dry out, and crumble away and the outer level of the skin begins to flake. Depending upon the severity, the condition can result in redness and scaling. Topical application of cholesterol effectively soothes and plumps up dry skin. Cholesterol decreases with age, so it may be an important component of topical treatments to protect the skin in older individuals.

Food and Herbal Agents That Slow Aging

A number of related plant-derived products prevent aging by a variety of mechanisms, including absorbing free radicals that lead to damage from such activities as sun exposure. Some of these products also reduce inflammation, increase collagen production, and activate genes that produce products to slow aging or increase antioxidant activity; a few of these extracts are discussed below:

- **Soy extracts** contain flavonoids that have both hormonal and collagen-stimulating effects. One of those is an "isoflavone" (a plant-derived compound that acts similarly to estrogen in the human body) named Genistein, which has antioxidant, anti-inflammatory, and phytoestrogen properties that help aging skin. Studies have shown that, over a prolonged period, oral soy isoflavones reduce wrinkling and thicken skin. Since these compounds are similar to estrogen, which has a similar anti-aging effect, this would be expected. They are especially useful in post-menopausal women who have lowered amounts of estrogen production as well as skin aging changes, whether or not they are from years of sun exposure and other oxidative stresses such as cigarette smoke exposure or from the natural aging process. Soy oil washes may slow down destruction of the collagen that accompanies aging. People with estrogen-sensitive tumors should avoid large applications of these products.

- **Resveratrol** is the well-known polyphenol compound from red wine that has a number of antioxidant properties. Its main sources are red grapes and Japanese knotwood root (Polygonium sp). It protects against sun damage, quenches free radicals produced by sun damage, reduces the inflammation from sun damage, and activates genes that increase antioxidant activity in the cells of the skin. Studies in mice show powerful antioxidant effect in protecting the skin against UV light exposure. Studies in irradiated skin of humans show improved thickening of the skin, and reduction of redness and other changes associated with aging, as well as a reduction in the level of enzymes that destroy the collagen and lead to aging. Other similar light-induced harmful body chemicals were also noted to be reduced. Other studies show that it has protective effects against the formation of skin cancers. Resveratrol has protective effects on the genetic material (DNA) of the cells that mimics the longevity effects of reduced calorie intake. Our genetic material has a limited number of caps, called telomeres, some of which are lost with each cell division. Resveratrol has been reported to help reduce the loss of telomeres, and thus slow aging of the cells. It might seem logical to use Resveratrol as part of a sunscreen or other topical application to reduce aging from sun damage; however, resveratrol is rapidly broken down in the body which means, as with any other sunscreen, it must be swallowed or applied regularly to maintain its effects. The type of formulation used may play a big role in its effectiveness and be difficult to evaluate by the consumer. It has potential benefits on aged skin, which might mean that the effects would be more dramatic in those who have been over rather than under fed. Also, since it is a phytoestrogen, large amounts of this product could be contra-indicated in those with estrogen-sensitive cancers such as breast or prostate cancer. Otherwise, no adverse effects are known to be associated with application of this product.

- **Green tea** contains flavonoids that have sun-protective, antioxidant effects that also help prevent inflammation and skin cancer. One of these phytochemicals is Epigallocatechin gallate, or EGCG—one of the most studied components of green tea, which has been incorporated into various products to protect the skin. Green tea extracts have also been shown to help prevent skin cancer initiated by light exposure. Green tea extract-containing products help protect against ongoing sun exposure, as well as past sun damage. One study showed that green tea extract, plus lotus, improved scaling, roughness, and wrinkling in healthy men.

Rarely, topical green tea will have a mild irritant effect. It is unlikely that the caffeine-like product in green tea extracts will be sufficient to affect those highly sensitive to coffee. The tannins in green tea extract may be drying for some people. Some people are concerned that green tea takes up and contains extra fluoride, so you may want to explore the fluoride levels in your green tea product, and use caution if you have elevated fluoride levels or if you have low thyroid activity (which could result from fluoride competing with iodide for binding onto your thyroid). Test tube experiments show that large doses of green tea extracts inhibit an enzyme related to the B-vitamin "folate" that is responsible for DNA production (dihydrofolate reductase), so that large amounts of green tea during pregnancy in mice leads to neural tube defects. This is not just a warning for mice. People who are deficient in folate or folic acid, or who have genetic defects related to the enzyme mentioned should use caution in applying large amounts of this product, as should pregnant women.

- **Curcumin,** the best known component of the yellow spice turmeric, has a number of protective effects on the skin. We now know that it acts as an antioxidant largely because of its epigenetic effects of binding to the DNA and activating antioxidant and other protective effects in the cells of the skin. Because of its intense yellow staining, ordinary curcumin is not easily used as a topical anti-aging cosmeceutical. There are colorless compounds derived from Curcumin that are incorporated into topical products. It is helpful in products that are designed for people whose skin aging has a component of inflammation, marked by redness and rapid degeneration of the skin elasticity.

- **Aloe vera** is known by many people for its healing effects on burns. It also has calming effects on inflammation of the skin, and is often used as a component in moisturizers, partly because of its soothing properties. The aloe from just inside the leaf may have a yellow color from compounds known as anthraquinones. This yellow portion can be a photosensitizer for some people, so caution should be used if you apply it and go out in the sun. Aloe is mostly water, so unless it is mixed with oils to make a cream, it may be very drying when the pure product is applied to the skin. It is a good component of products used to treat burns.

- **Chamomile** has important protective effects for irritated skin. It has anti-inflammatory effects, and has been shown to be the equivalent of 0.25 percent hydrocortisone in one study. It also has antimicrobial effects against common skin bacteria such as Staph (Staphylococcus aureus). Hence, it is a good first aid application for minor skin irritations. For some people who are very sensitive to herbs, it has a mild sleep-inducing effect, especially when applied to areas of thin skin such as the eyelids. Therefore, it may be a good nighttime application for people with mildly irritated skin who also need a little help relaxing and going to sleep. Chamomile should not be used by people who are allergic to other plants of the Compositae family, which includes such plants as ragweed, goldenrod, chrysanthemum, marigold, and sunflower. And people who are highly sensitive to the sleep-inducing effects should not apply massive amounts to their face before driving.

Minerals

- **Zinc salts** are well known for their healing effects on the skin. White zinc oxide ointment is familiar as both a protector for irritated baby bottoms, and as a coating to protect the nose from sunburns. The first time I investigated the role of zinc as a helper (cofactor) for enzymes in the body, I found 70 different enzymatic reactions in which zinc was necessary for function. The current number of enzymes now recognized to require zinc is over 200, and growing. It is no wonder that this mineral is helpful in keeping the skin healthy. It is important in the enzymes that play a role in wound healing and in remodeling of damaged skin. It is probably the safest mineral to use as a sunscreen component because it not only helps protect against sun radiation, but has many other beneficial effects on the skin and body as well. An individual who is especially low in copper in the body and skin might not benefit from zinc applications, because zinc can compete with copper for uptake into the cells.

- **Copper** is a component of one of the critical enzymes responsible for the formation of the pigment in the cell, known as melanin. It also is important in the enzymes that give the skin its strength and elasticity via collagen and elastin. A particular copper peptide, tripeptide glycyl-L-histidyl-L-lysine (GHK), marketed for improving aging, has been formulated for effects of the peptide and perhaps better penetration into the skin. A number of effects have been claimed for this combination product that go far beyond the supplying of copper for antioxidant properties and as a cofactor for synthesis of elastin. Some of these effects are attributed to the peptide itself, including gene regulation and stimulation of blood vessel growth. Studies on skin fibroblasts in the test tube show that copper itself increases tissue information factors whose loss is associated with aging (transforming growth factor-[TGF-] and vascular endothelial growth factor [VEGF]).

Some individuals experience improvement of scars and wrinkles from copper tripeptides and others are unhappy with its results. Not enough information is available to determine who is likely to benefit and who is likely to get worse. It may be that someone who is copper-deficient would be more likely to benefit. That individual would probably not have copper plumbing in their house or have copper pots, and might take zinc supplements regularly, which would reduce the absorption of copper. On the other hand, someone with copper plumbing might be more likely to already have sufficient or excess supplies of copper, especially if they cook with hot water from the tap (which would have higher amounts of copper dissolved in it).

Individual Specificity

People often wonder whether they will get similar results with a new anti-aging product as they see in the photos, advertisements, or their friends' faces. Even if the product has effect, the photos are accurate, and the data is not manipulated, individual uniqueness makes a big difference in the results achieved. If you examine the data from cosmeceutical studies, you will find that some people get outstanding improvements while others hardly change. It is important to remember that individuals differ in their genetic and environmental strengths and weaknesses, and respond differently to applications of natural and chemical products. For instance, one person could have wrinkles aggravated by a deficiency of a particular mineral such as copper. In that case, application of a product that contains an absorbable form of copper might produce a much greater improvement in her wrinkles than on someone else's. Throwing a lot of different herbs and nutrients into a cream could help some people, but in others, cause allergy or inactivate key ingredients within the products. You would think that if you add ten ingredients together and they each make a ten percent improvement in the skin, the whole product should result in more than a ten percent improvement; however, that is not always the case.

Several years ago I was asked to evaluate the results of a study on a combination cosmeceutical from a well-established manufacturer. The various ingredients had been well chosen for their effectiveness in slowing aging by a wide variety of different mechanisms. Proof of that was provided by the manufacturers of each of the main components in a three-inch binder describing the studies and the degree of improvement of various parameters of aging (such as a wrinkle index) using each compound, as well as basic studies on the mechanism of such improvement. Most fascinating to me was that many of the ingredients were reported to have greater anti-aging effects (such as reduction of "crow's feet") separately than in the final combination used, which gave, at best, an eight percent average improvement. That means that each component, when taken separately, produced a greater degree of improvement than the combination product. If we assume that all, or even most of the component manufacturers' data was accurate, we can only guess that something went wrong when "the right stuff" was put together. There may have been chemical interactions rendering the components ineffective, or the interactions in complex biochemical processes in the cells may have interfered with one another (thinking back, some of the chemical interactions that cancelled each other's benefits could have been prevented by coating the active ingredients by a process known as "microencapsulation": that is, placing a molecular coating over the chemical so that it went to the right place in the cell, did not interfere with other chemicals, or was released at the proper time and in the proper sequence). This demonstrates that simply because a product has a list of seemingly impressive ingredients, doesn't mean that it's going to be the most effective treatment for you and your unique makeup.

Designing cosmeceutical products is challenging because of the factors and variations mentioned above. Test tube evaluations of particular functions, such as antioxidant support, support of normal cell growth and collagen formation, and presence of healthy skin-related signaling molecules are all used to check the effectiveness of individual products and formulations. All of these studies, plus trial and error and past experience, help in the art of combining cosmeceuticals. It is completely unrealistic to do large studies on all the possible combinations of active ingredients, so actual testing on a group of people large enough to give statistically reliable results is only done on the final product, which is put together from all the supporting information mentioned above. This means that the only way to determine if a product will work for you is to try it yourself for a period of time to see if it is really helpful. This discussion is not meant to discourage you from using cosmeceuticals for beauty and reducing the effects of aging; rather, it is to inform you about the reality of the situation so that you can better interpret manufacturers' claims and choose which products may work best for you.

The Botox Option

If you have deep muscular wrinkles of the brow, the current dermatologic treatment attests to the power of the underlying process that forms these wrinkles. That treatment involves injecting botulism toxin, one of the most powerful toxins known to man, into the muscles that are contracting and forming the crease. It causes the muscle to relax for half a year or more, flattening the brow crease. It certainly is an option, but a radical one. It should give you some perspective on how toxic the crease-causing negative emotions can be, and how much effort is required to change them.

The Path to Inner Beauty

Some years ago, I met the distributor of an elite natural cosmetic company. The company sent an esthetician to my office to do herbal facials on a few of my patients. The first two women came from their facials happy and relaxed, even glowing slightly. The esthetician was massaging and relaxing patients' facial muscles using essential oils that balanced their temperament, as well as using a few of the "elite" products. One woman in particular, Mary, never seemed to be a happy person when I saw her, and most likely as a result, never appeared especially attractive. Indeed, just like her dour mood, her appearance was rather dour, too, from her clothing to her speech. Other than vaguely noticing the rather depressive, worn feeling I got whenever Mary walked into the office, I had never made much of the connection between her demeanor and her appearance.

However, when Mary came back from her facial massage with well-chosen oils and quality products, I could hardly believe my eyes! She emerged a beautiful woman, with all the tension I had seen in her face gone. I never suspected that such an attractive face lay beneath all that stress. I wished that I had before and after photos; I could have sold anything associated with that improvement. She was relaxed and very happy about the change.

More and more, I see the lines on people's faces from the expressions they make over and over. For instance, the repeated brow-furrowing from anger leaves creases between the eyes. Muscle development and furrows in the dermal collagen contribute to all of this. These are the very creases that call for Botox to relax, and later for dermal fillers to smooth them out.

Let me be more specific. I see a number of rather attractive female patients who develop deep creases between their eyebrows related to muscles conveying facial expressions of anger. I suspect some of these women have spent their lives being hit upon so regularly that they wear the creases caused by repeating the same angry expression over and over again for years. Life circumstances and coping difficulties may cause creases in others.

There are other women who start out with naturally beautiful features who seem to expect that the world ought to treat them specially all the time (as some men have done some of the time) and their anger at not getting that sort of special care comes through with the same sort of creases. Some of these women look fine when they are relaxed, but show the creases and expressions of that hard and angry side whenever they become animated or upset. These are many of the same women who get Botox injections and injections of fillers in the creases to erase the facial expressions of anger that seethe out of them at the slightest provocation. Other women with less striking features appear attractive because their smiles come straight from their hearts.

A big part of beauty starts with one's inner feelings and the reactions they lead to. Natural beauty comes from a beautiful response to the world around you. Notice the change in the appearance of people you are with between gloom, tension, or anger, and true joy. Look at yourself in a mirror in these different conditions. Which *you* is more attractive?

Having a skilled facial massage, feeling really relaxed and good about yourself, using essential oils to balance out your emotions, all put you back in touch with your true beautiful self. Even though one beauty editor made me remove a point about inner feelings and beauty from a brief article on beauty tips, as she deemed it too unsophisticated, I must state the truth here. The most important single thing you can do to be more beautiful is to get in touch with your happiness, and quietly let it radiate from your being through your smile.

When I was a child, I would sometimes get angry and walk around with a sour expression on my face. My mother chided me saying, "I hope a cold wind freezes that expression on your face so that you have to look at it forever in the mirror." I learned the grain of truth in what she said as I got older and met angry people who showed, even when relaxed, deep creases between their eyebrows. It appeared that the repetitive use of the same muscles over years, producing the same lines over and over again, began to result in permanent furrows. I have seen these furrows exaggerated in Japanese prints of fierce warriors. I have also noticed the smile lines and pleasing wrinkles in pictures of Mother Teresa or paintings of Native American Elders that seem to come from repeated expressions of peace, happiness, and inner joy. The muscles of expression enlarge and the creases form much like when we repeatedly fold a fabric in the same direction. This is all magnified by muscular repetition of the same facial expressions out of habitual experience of the same emotions.

The first step in lessening these lines and creases is to identify when you are making those repeated scowls and other unattractive facial expressions. Use a pocket mirror to peek at what faces you are making while you are on the phone or when you feel various emotions coming up. Ask your friends or family to let you know when you have the most lines in your face. These creases don't only come from negative emotions. I often see otherwise attractive people who habitually crunch up their brow to emphasize their concern, when the caring reflected in their speech would more than suffice. Eight hours a day of working and listening and more "caring" with the brow at home, and it's not surprising that these furrows can become prominent even if you are in your 30s. It is helpful to remember that others can really feel the help you are giving, and that if you simply devote that extra brow-creasing energy to listening and responding, your effect will be greater. Smiling can lead to more pleasing creases. I am not arguing here to keep a poker face and to stuff your emotions down inside behind a faint, put-on smile, but rather to become aware of what emotions are repeatedly being expressed on your face and what their source is.

Let's explore the steps you can take when you identify the emotion you are feeling, using anger as an example. If you see furrows of anger between your eyebrows, find out why you are always so angry. Does everything bring up some deep-seated anger from the past, or does it seem that life always deals you a bad hand? Check and see if you appreciate the good things you do have in your life. Are you contributing in any way to the issues that make you angry? When you think about what triggers your anger, is there some underlying belief about how you should be treated that justifies your anger? Sometimes, just thinking about that belief will be enough to help you see that it was simply something you assumed to be true. When you let it go, all the anger that it justified unblocks and flows away as if you cleared a log jam from a river. Physical exercise can help remove the last remains of the hormones and chemical signals released by that anger from your system.

We often choose to assuage our anger by giving in to "pleasures" such as overeating. How many times will we choose to have the same superficial pleasure and then "pay for it" afterwards? After a certain number of times of paying for the same pleasure with pain, we have got to admit that there must be something very wrong going on underneath for us to make a bad choice over and over. After we get over the excuses that it's what we like, or that we have a right to it, or others can do it without problems, we have to face what it is doing to us, and what it might be leading to. Ignorance is only an excuse until our awareness gets touched by how we feel, what we read, or what a friend may say (*see Illustration page 115*).

The hardest pain cycles are the ones we are not really completely aware of, stuck in our unconscious minds. Think of a time when some little thing that a family member did made you screaming angry. Looking back at it: there is no way that leaving the seat up on the toilet (or whatever it was) deserved that kind of response, so there must have been some underlying cause for your outburst. A lot of "stuff" may be coming from your unconscious mind from the reactivation of old painful issues that were never fully faced and released.

Some people can bring this unconscious stuff to mind just by watching how they are behaving. Looking at yourself in a mirror, seeing what kind of expression is on your face, listening to your tone of voice, and what effect you have on others is a start. Then think about why you are reacting with the emotions you expressed. When you notice how you are reacting and can identify the emotion, you can begin to think about why you are angry (or whatever emotion may be involved).

Writing down your dreams is another source of clues. They may emerge during meditation, when you quiet your mind. A good psychotherapist can expose these emotions, often by having you watch them surface in your interactions with others. Sometimes, experiencing these emotions and releasing them seems more than is rationally possible. In this case, you must find a way to ask the help of the Great Healer, by whatever Name you prefer and whatever method of asking you are comfortable using. For many, this means praying to God, or asking their angels or guides to help them find the path. It can also mean enlisting the help of friends, family, support groups, and therapists. When the path is clear, it means doing whatever it takes to change a habit that is dragging you, your health, and your appearance down with it. Both paths are always open, and you have a choice.

If all of this doesn't help enough, it may be time to enter a path of healing of your anger and inner torments. Sometimes this means changing a set of external circumstances that are bad enough to make a saint scream. Reading, journaling, and sharing with close friends may help. Twelve-Step groups and Co-Counseling can be of therapeutic benefit if you can afford the time but not the money. Forgiving and releasing long-carried resentments and making a list of all the gifts in life you have to appreciate can release anger and give you a fresh perspective on life. If none of this is sufficient to help deal with the underlying feelings and issues you uncover, it's time to consider working them out through some form of therapeutic relationship. The cost can be justified not just by the furrows it smooths, but by the underlying radiance it allows to come back into your life.

Illustration
"Stuffing" Emotions

Why do we eat things that aren't good for us? Sometimes, we are fully aware of painful emotions such as anger or fear, or we can clearly see their effects on our thoughts or behavior, but we seem unable to change them. Other times, painful emotions may lurk beneath the surface of our awareness, producing a vague feeling of discomfort that won't go away. Some of us learn to bury that feeling by stuffing ourselves with "comfort food," or by engaging in some other addictive behavior that blots out the pain. The "stuffing" and its side-effects will linger until the pain underneath is worked through, and that's when nutritional balance can flow again naturally.

Stuffing emotional pain

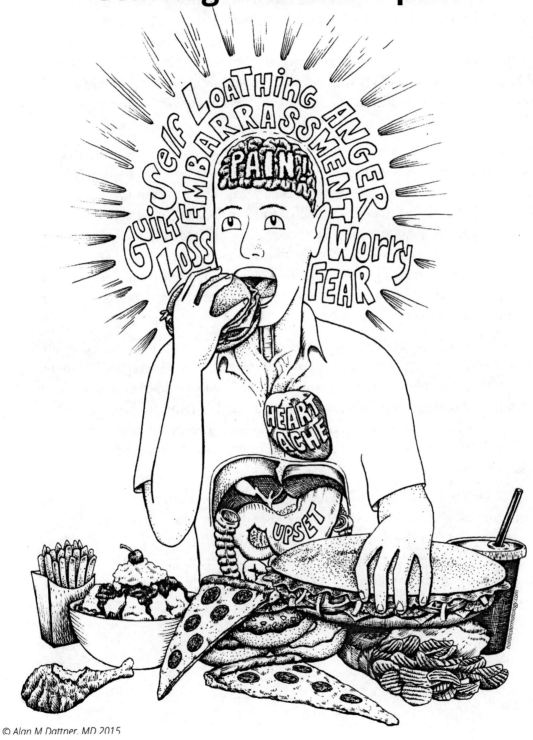

© Alan M Dattner, MD 2015

Healing Your Anger

If you can't afford professional help, it may be that a close friend is all you need. When I take lunchtime walks with a close friend, or share from the heart over the phone, I make sure that I am there to listen and give honest feedback to them in equal time. When my perspective or self interest influences my response, I do my best to say so and get that out in the open, along with my opinion. And I call my friends out on their biases or take their advice cautiously when self-interest clouds their perspective. And I hope that they will do the same for me.

A recent patient reminded me of the old adage that true beauty comes from the inside. Surprised at how young she looked, I inquired beyond her face cream technique, which seemed insufficient to explain her youthful appearance. I found that she also meditated regularly during the day, and was involved in a multifaceted spiritual path that she described with enthusiasm and joy. When I heard all this, the mystery was solved; all of that radiance simply bubbled up to the surface of her face from the inside. The process of bringing yourself back to a state of inner calm, joy, and clarity can have a dramatic effect on improving your appearance and the creases that you show.

I recently questioned a woman whom I originally mistook for the daughter of an attendee at a 60s high school reunion. She used sunscreen regularly, avoided sun, did exercises to tighten and relax her mouth and tighten her neck, and always tried to find something good in each day. This further reinforced my impression that proper exercising of the facial muscles, through expression of emotion or conscious exercise over a long period of time, enhances beauty and maintains a youthful appearance.

Dr. Deepak Chopra has shown us that we feel as young as we choose to feel. He mentions a study in which Baby Boomers were put into an environment that mimicked their high school days. They were played music from high school, etc., and the people in the study actually began to feel younger. We respond to cues in our environment to tell us how to feel, but we can also create those cues internally.

Summary

Many of the changes we associate with aging are accelerated by damage from sunlight, accumulation of AGE's oxidative damage and toxins, and inflammation from allergy and accumulation of the wrong fatty acids. We can slow what we see as aging by preventing or repairing this sort of damage. Remember that the expressions of inner joy, health, and rested well-being make many people look more attractive than even Botox or plastic surgery can accomplish. Focus on total health. Aside from the various lotions that are reported to be beneficial in some associated regard, the overall perspective and methods in this book will provide a path to keep your skin looking younger from the inside out.

CHAPTER 9
TAKING CARE OF YOUR SKIN HOLISTICALLY

Imagine a house whose shingles keep its inhabitant dry and warm. Imagine that these shingles fall off as new shingles grow from underneath. Imagine also that it comes complete with roofing cement to make a good barrier. If a falling branch should create a tear or hole, the roof can repair itself. It can also warn suspected intruders to stay away by putting out an obnoxious odor. If the intruders are small, information is brought to a local police station where they are identified and a response is initiated. If a large intruder does get in, signals are sent to the central intelligence authority. If the house gets too hot, it could wet the roof and cool it off by evaporation. The outside of the house could last for 50 to 80 years with a little care, but without a paint job or replacement.

Your skin is the house you live in, having all the features of the imaginary house above. It is an amazing series of layers that grow out and develop constantly. The layers of the skin shelter you from the elements, then fall off as new layers grow from underneath. Just as our imagined roof, the skin has a remarkable ability to repair itself. If "intruders" such as bacteria and other organisms should gain entry, sentinel cells called "Langerhans" cells pick up intruder material and bring it back to the lymph nodes for identification and preparation of white cells to attack. If the body gets too hot, millions of glands under the skin produce sweat, which seeps from tiny holes called pores; the body cools down when the sweat evaporates. Apocrine glands under the arms put out a bad odor when you are anxious or facing danger.

If you had an amazing house whose outside took care of itself as well as our skin takes care of us, wouldn't you want to know as much as possible about what you can do to make it function efficiently and last as long as possible?

In this chapter, I am going to share some simple secrets of skin care that might improve the appearance of your entire skin over a lifetime, and cost no more than taking the effort to put some good habits into place on a regular basis. If you ever doubted the wisdom of spending the money to buy this book or taking the time to read it, you will look back on the value of this chapter's secrets as being worth the price a hundred times over.

Washing

The skin may not need replacement, but it does need care, and the most fundamental type of care is washing. There are certain areas of the skin that need to be washed more often than others. Your hands touch so many things during the course of a day that they need to be cleaned often to prevent contaminating yourself or others. Your face is exposed to the elements and may get dirty or oily, so it should be cleaned once, twice, or even three times per day. Underarms develop odor and need to be washed daily (or more) if you do not use deodorant. The groin and buttocks area may also need to be cleaned daily, or more often.

However, there are many areas of the skin that do not really need to be cleaned each day. We have become accustomed to the convenience and luxury of hot running water and a shower before work in this country, but this was by no means the way our ancestors lived. It is cleansing, convenient, awakening, helpful for sore muscles, and a nice way to start the day or wash off the dirt from work; but for many people, especially in the winter, daily bathing is just too drying. It washes off the skin's oils, and it washes off the salts that bind water in the skin. If you have ever spent too much time with your hands in and out of water at the sink, you know the "chapped" feeling that occurs when your hands become too dry. The same thing happens to the rest of your skin when you bathe too much.

Each person has to choose how much to bathe based on a series of factors. The drier the air outside is, such as when the temperature and humidity drop during the winter, the less bathing your skin will tolerate. The hotter and more humid it is, the more you will want to bathe and the frequency will cause less risk of drying your skin. If you sweat a lot, exercise, have more body odor, work around dust, dirt, or toxic materials, you will probably want to bathe more. People with oily skin can tolerate more bathing. People with dry skin may not be able to tolerate the amount of bathing they reasonably think they need.

Soaps

A true soap is a combination of an alkali (a substance that forms a salt when mixed with an acid) with an oil or fat. As a result, soaps have a high "pH"; that is, they are very alkaline. The skin does best being more acidic, toward a neutral pH, than true soaps offer, so good rinsing is important. Many people find excessive use of true soaps too irritating. Castile soaps use oil instead of a solid fat. A good natural soap will use pure vegetable oils such as olive, coconut, safflower, or sesame (saturated and rancid animal fat may be used in poor quality soaps). Some brands include powerful essential oils that give a fresh feeling, but may aggravate people who are allergic to the fragrance used. I prefer soaps without a fragrance or essential oil added.

Syndets, Anyone?

Most commercially available cleansing bars that we call soap today are really not soaps, but are **syn**thetic **de**tergents, referred to as syndets. They allow a more neutral pH. Many of them have extra oil or fat added to give a moisturizing effect. Dove® bars, which were launched in 1955, were the first syndet bars produced. Some of the syndets have antibacterial substances to "keep you smelling fresh all day" by killing the bacteria that cause odor to develop under your arms. In the 1970s, some of those substances also caused some people to develop allergies when exposed to the sun. Those "photosensitizing" anti-bacterials have supposedly been banned and removed, but it is an issue to keep in mind when traveling or using old anti-bacterial or deodorant soap.

Bath oils

The idea of using a bath oil is that when you are all wet in the tub, you have an oil floating on the top of the water. When you get up, the oil coats you all over as you move through it. I prefer a natural vegetable oil to the mineral oil products often marketed. Some bath oils have a detergent added so that they disperse better in the water.

Moisturizers

Some of the oil that has been removed by bathing can be replaced by applying moisturizers to the skin. Creams contain both water, to hydrate the skin, and oils, to seal that moisture in. Most also contain "humectants," which hold water in the skin. Ointments and oils must be used on wet skin to seal that water in. Otherwise, unless you sweat, your skin will still be and feel dry. Natural products make sense because they tend to be more nourishing and less harmful than synthetics. Remember that some of these products are actually entering your skin, so it is best to use products you don't mind having inside your body. Petroleum products, such as petroleum jelly and mineral oil, tend to be thicker and stay on the body longer, sealing moisture in the skin longer, in some people.

Creams are much more pleasing to use, but they bring up another issue. Creams (which are mixtures of oil and water) usually have to be held together by some ingredient that acts as a detergent. Oil and water mixes are much more prone to bacteria or fungus growing in them, so preservatives have to be added to prevent this. These preservatives may cause low-grade allergic reactions, or have other influences such as on the body's hormones or chemistry. Some of the oils and fats used commercially have a faintly unpleasant smell or color, so fragrances and coloring agents are added to make them more pleasing. And a variety of other synthetic products are added to make them penetrate better and feel and look more pleasing. The biggest problem with applying lotions and creams to moisturize your skin is that some of these various ingredients can cause allergic reactions, especially if they are put on already irritated or inflamed skin.

Sometimes it takes industrial chemistry detective work to identify what chemically-related substances in the cream you're using may be causing an allergic reaction. For instance, formaldehyde chemicals are present in Stay-pressed cotton clothing, sized cotton, plywood, pressboard, and resins (including Melamine), to name a few. Related aldehydes de-gas (escape into the air) from a variety of synthetic products including carpets, automobile interiors, wallpaper, and upholstery. People with rashes (and even physicians) sometimes forget that the same chemical that caused an allergy to one cream may be released by preservatives with different names in a substitute cream. Changing to a different cream may not help, because so many of the same fragrances, detergents, smoothing agents, preservatives, and colors turn up in different products with different names. So creams can be helpful at first, but backfire later, causing an allergic reaction and more inflammation. For that reason, I am including here a short list of preservative chemicals that keep bacteria from growing in creams by releasing formaldehyde (the chemical name for these products may be written differently for some):

Formaldehyde releasers:

- Quaternium-15
- Imidazolidinyl urea (Germail 115)
- Diazolidinyl urea (Germall II)
- DMDM hydantoin (Glydant)
- Tris (hydroxymethyl) nitromethane (Tris Nitro)
- Hydroxymethylglycinate (Suttocide A)

Other types of synthetic preservatives that do not release formaldehyde include benzyl alcohol, Phenoxyethanol, and sodium EDTA.

As far as skin applications go, "there is no free lunch." You can use oils and ointments applied to wet skin to seal in moisture. They are much less elegant than creams and lotions because they require wetting the skin, and they are greasy. Creams are mixtures of oil and water, and will grow bacteria and mold if they are not kept in the refrigerator or mixed with preservatives. You have to choose your preservatives wisely, because some types may cause allergy, including essential oils and fragrances. Over the years, significant amounts of Parabens (chemical compounds used as preservatives) can accumulate in your body from daily widespread use, and can potentially disrupt your hormones by mimicking estrogen and contribute to abnormalities and even possibly to cancer. Direct cause has not been proven, but the suspicion remains. Chemicals in cosmetics enter the body through the skin, so they can affect the body.

Essential oils from herbs kill microbes and can also be used as preservatives. Remember that herbs are weeds, and some people are allergic to the chemicals in herbs, as well. They may be far safer than synthetics, but the risk of aggravation remains. If you have a persistent rash, you have to know what you are putting onto your skin. That is not always so easy when you only see the word "fragrance" on your container of hand or body cream, and it does not tell you which fragrances were mixed into the product. It is also difficult because products in this country can be labeled "scent-free" yet and still include what is known as a masking fragrance, which hides the odor of the product. Not until the labeling laws catch up to the product manufacturers will people really know what might be aggravating them in their skin creams. Some of the natural product manufacturers may follow a higher standard, and tell you what is in their creams, so this may be another reason to make the more expensive choice.

A good dermatologist familiar with contact sensitivity should be able to help you choose the creams and oils most appropriate for you. You may also have to do some learning and detective work yourself to find out what is causing your problem, and help you avoid rash circumstances.

Using oils to which you have not been previously exposed, such as jojoba oil or shea butter, may be helpful because you are less likely to already be allergic to them. Oils that cut down inflammation such as vitamin E, or omga-3 oils, fish oil, and flax oil may nourish the skin and even provide some anti-inflammatory effects. I am always concerned that people who already have inflamed skin may develop an allergy to these important oils when they are applied to that inflamed area. The oils are too important as internal anti-inflammatory substances to take a chance on developing an allergy to them, making them useless as anti-inflammatory treatments, so I avoid applying them topically.

Skin Brushing

The skin needs touch, and it needs stimulation, just as any other organ of the body. Tiny channels called "lymphatics" carry fluid from the cells in the skin and other organs back to where they can re-enter the blood. These channels do not have the thick muscular walls that arteries or veins have, and are much harder to see on a biopsy than the tiniest blood vessels, known as capillaries. They seem to need a little help from gravity or from gentle pressure to move the lymph fluid along.

There are also nerve endings in the skin that send messages back to the brain. There are numerous ways in which the effects of every kind of manipulation of the skin can cause a response. It has been demonstrated that repeated touching, rubbing, or squeezing of the skin thickens the skin and causes the formation or enlargement of structures such as oil glands and hair follicles. So a part of the skin that is regularly touched and squeezed may become thicker and develop more hair than the surrounding area.

On that basis, a gentler, more systematic rubbing or brushing of the skin may help keep the skin from becoming thinner with age. Although much less commonly recommended than bathing, a number of people have advocated skin brushing over the years, especially in the alternative medicine world. Sometimes this method is called dry brushing or air brushing. It consists of using a soft natural bristle brush with gentle strokes in a particular direction. Some brush toward a point near the navel, which overlies the central collecting cistern for the lymph channels from the body, known as the Cisterna Chili. From here, the Thoracic Duct brings the lymph up to return to the circulation, emptying into a vein underneath the left collarbone. Of course, you would not want to brush over a suspected skin cancer, so you should have your skin checked regularly if you do this practice.

If you have a problem with fluid accumulation in the skin, such as lymphedema (partial blockage of the lymphatics causing swelling) after breast removal surgery, you probably want to seek out the best lymphatic massage therapists available. There are a number of different schools of lymphatic massage, each with their own exacting techniques. Vodder massage is a method of manual lymph drainage that very gently cleanses the body, reduces swelling, and strengthens the immune system. Electronic devices are also used. For people with lymphedema, drainage by an expert skilled in specific techniques can make a huge difference. For the average person, light brushing may stimulate the flow of lymph, "awaken" the skin, thicken it, and actually keep it from getting thin (atrophying) with age. Light touch actually "milks" the lymphatic fluid through the lymphatic channels back to the lymph nodes, and eventually back to the central collecting system. From there it travels through the thoracic duct, and re-enters the veins underneath the left collar bone. There is some evidence that the direction of tugging on the fibroblasts, the cells that make collagen, influences the growth of these cells. So keeping some tension on these cells with brushing may keep this layer tight. This may be why, once the skin becomes lax, it seems to fall apart rapidly. Although the actual effects of skin brushing remain unproven, I think there is enough evidence to recommend it as a morning ritual to stimulate the skin and perhaps even get the lymphatic flow moving.

Most people benefit from some kind of fairly regular brushing. You can use a soft brush on a long handle, gently brushing your skin all over toward your navel, when you awaken in the morning and are undressed. If you do not have a brush handy, rubbing with a Turkish towel will have a similar effect in "waking up" your skin. Notice that after even a few strokes, your skin tingles and feels more alive. Your skin deserves to be awakened in the morning just like the rest of you. If you have a skin condition, you should avoid brushing over that area unless you have checked this out with your dermatologist or doctor.

Picking and scratching

This probably seems like the last thing you would find on a list of recommended skin care practices. Well, it is **not recommended**, but it is so common and so hushed up that I feel it must be discussed openly. For many people with skin conditions, the damage to appearance caused by picking at the blemishes is greater than by the disease process itself. It becomes a habit and then an addiction, often well beyond the original stimulus such as the itching it counteracted. For some, despite the damage and scarring it causes on the skin, it is as hard a habit to break as cigarette or heroin addiction. Whether it is an itch or a new acne pimple, the fingernails go on automatic pilot and start touching or squeezing, creating a new blemish or aggravating an old one. Of course, the answer is simple: stop scratching or picking and substitute a new habit, such as applying a therapeutic cream. But the answer is not easy, and you may need support and hard work to slowly shift this pattern. That support can come from your family, a therapist, or a support group experienced in breaking addiction patterns.

One way to break the habit, when you notice yourself "digging" at your skin, is to pause, take a four-second deep breath, and gently remove your fingers and your attention from the area being attacked. Take a few more slow breaths and just let yourself become aware of any conflicts that might be picking at your emotions. Sometimes, becoming aware of what is bothering you and letting it go with a few deep breaths can release the pressure to pick. You will have to be gentle and forgiving with yourself, as you release this habit again and again, only to find it still returns and needs to be dropped another time. With persistence and, if needed, proper emotional support, you can succeed in reducing this habit over time.

Summary

This chapter is a brief description of how to take care of normal skin with a natural perspective, focusing on treatment from the outside. Some conditions require other external treatments. This book focuses on internal treatment of skin conditions, which can be enhanced by treatment of the underlying issues inside the body. If you develop good regular habits for taking care of your skin, its appearance and function will be better now and over time.

CHAPTER 10

A RAISIN IN THE SUN: SUNBURNED AND PREMATURELY AGED

Let me introduce you to Giselle, an attractive natural blond who enjoyed being out in the sun. She spent all her summers with her friends at the beach getting as much of a tan as her pale skin would allow. When she grew up, living the charmed life of a vibrant young woman, she and several close friends motored their yacht down to the coast of Mexico and spent three years living in a tropical paradise. Even with the use of a little sun protection from time to time, she got sunburned regularly, and often had a red nose or red skin to show for her adventures.

When she came to see me, she had several rough red spots on her face and other sun-exposed areas, which were pre-cancers from the sun, known as "actinic keratoses." These are not dangerous, but are a sign of too much sun and are more common on people in their 70s than young women in their 30s. All over the areas where the sun had touched, she also had splotches of brown color, patchy enlarged fine veins, and wrinkling, all characteristic of solar aging. More disturbing was a somewhat blackish spot with irregular pigmentation, which she pointed out to me. I biopsied it, taking care to remove the entire lesion. Sure enough, it was a malignant melanoma. She agreed to have a wider excision done around the biopsied area, to be sure that we removed all of it.

Giselle's skin was a few decades older than she was. This made it hard for her to go safely about her usual life, because she still really enjoyed outdoor sports, and her skin had already had its limit of sun. And she already had a potentially fatal skin cancer, melanoma, which behaves much more aggressively than the more common sun-induced skin cancers. Having one melanoma makes it more likely to develop another if the same sun damage persists.

This may sound like a more extreme case, but remember that the incidence of melanoma is rising so rapidly that one out of forty-nine people are now expected to develop melanoma in their lifetimes.

The Sun and Aging

You may be protesting before you even start to read this, thinking "What can I do about the exposure I got in the past?" "I'm good looking, but with a tan and my white dress, I'm a real knockout." "My favorite thing in the world is to be outside at the beach, swimming and running to get exercise, or lying in the sand basking in the warmth of the sun and relaxing into Mother Earth. Don't even think about taking all this away from me!" To this I say, there are many paths, and some walk the fine line of compromise to meet conflicting needs and requirements. I cannot make the hard choices for you, but I can give you some vital information to make informed, sensible decisions amid a complex series of individual factors influencing your skin.

Let's be realistic. Excess solar damage, in the form of ultraviolet light, is the greatest cause of skin damage besides the natural aging process. Your likelihood of sun aging increases with the fairness of your skin color, as discussed in the next paragraph. Most of this damage comes from the sun, although UV lights, arc welding, radiation damage from high altitude, and other forms of radiation may contribute. But the skin has a certain amount of natural tolerance to sun damage. This is done by the re-positioning of pigment granules in the skin (known to dermatologists as immediate pigment darkening), and the production of pigment (tanning) known as melanin. We are also protected by a number of antioxidant systems within the body, and by antioxidants taken in with our food, both of which can be enhanced with proper supplementation. The key concept here is that if we stay within the capabilities of our own skin to darken slowly and over time to protect us, and within the capabilities of our skin to quench excessive free radicals and remain calm, we will be able to enjoy being outdoors, get some color, and not make our skin look wrinkled and old before its time. There are some important qualifications to this statement, and they will be the subject of this section.

The first characteristic to take into account is a combination of skin color and ease of tanning versus burning. You can tell most of this by looking at your hair and skin color. If you have blond hair and fair skin and burn easily, you probably fall into the category of most sun sensitive. A well-known dermatologist created a scale from I to VI to quickly classify people into categories of sun sensitivity, with category I being the most sensitive, and category VI (for people with brown-black skin) being the least sensitive. Ancestor analysis usually shows adaptation to climate and sun exposure conferred by skin color and ease of sun penetration through the skin. For instance, Celtic people from Ireland needed fair enough skin to make enough Vitamin D to keep from getting Rickets during the cloudy months or short cold days. In contrast, African people needed dark skin to protect them from the harsh rays of the sun near the equator, where it was too hot and uncomfortable to be covered up.

Sun Protection and Youthful Looking Skin

In a TV interview, I was once asked, impromptu, "What is the most important herb for sun protection?" Without thinking I answered, "Straw; you weave it into a hat and cover your head from the sun." Though my comment was greeted with laughter from the audience, it is no joke. Protection from excessive sun hitting your skin is still the best and most natural method of protecting your skin from burning and the harmful effects of sun exposure. That means staying out of the sun during the hours of 11:00 AM to 4:00 PM, when it is highest in the sky, using sun protective clothing when spending time outdoors, and staying in the shade when possible. The degree to which you must protect yourself from the sun depends on the amount of natural pigmentation you have in your skin, both inherited and from tanning.

Pros and Cons of Sun Exposure

Sun exposure has benefits and drawbacks. On the positive side, sun exposure activates production of Vitamin D, as well as some of the immune cells in the skin. Many people feel relaxed in the sun, meditate on the warmth, and enjoy getting a tan. There is a sense that tanning makes one look more attractive, and every young person wants to look the best they can.

Benefits of sun exposure include feelings of relaxation and well-being, vitamin D production, and enhancing immunity. However, as with so many things, there is an ideal amount of sun exposure beyond which the benefits become risks. Dr. Michael Holick, author of *The Vitamin D Solution*, suggests that getting about

10 minutes of sunshine a day facing both toward and away from the sun will produce sufficient vitamin D. Dr. Holick suffered academic reprisal for his views, as many dermatologists argue that you should take vitamin D orally and avoid the damage by the sun. Vitamin D is important not only for the absorption of calcium to build strong bones and to prevent osteopenia (bone loss not as severe as osteoporosis). It is also important for strengthening the immune system against everything from infection to cancer, and at the same time, protecting against overreaction of the immune system in autoimmune disorders.

Many people like the cosmetic effect of a suntan, an outward symbol of their sporty, outdoor nature. Some skin diseases, including psoriasis, eczema, acne, and some cases of vitiligo, may benefit from sun exposure. There is some sun protection provided by the increased melanin pigmentation that occurs in people chronically exposed to the sun. A proponent of sun exposure benefits, Dr. Johan Moan, of the Norwegian Institute for Cancer Research, also points out that sun exposure generates nitric oxide formation, which in turn opens up blood vessels to relax the cardiovascular system.

In recent years, there have been a number of studies that show mechanisms that moderate the damage potentially caused by light exposure of the skin. Molecules that increase the production of melanin are generated with sunshine, and some of these may offer immune protective effects. Furthermore, a number of studies have shown that increased exposure to ultraviolet light and its vitamin D generation lowered the incidence of 15 types of cancer.

On the other hand, dermatologist-researchers such as Dr. John Voorhees of the University of Michigan Medical School show data on destructive changes of the structure of the skin from even small doses of sunlight that are a fraction of the amount of sunlight needed to give the first signs of skin redness.

Too much sun exposure weakens immune cells in the skin. Nearly 40 years ago, in our laboratory at the NIH, we showed that UV light exposure weakens immune response as seen by the reduced ability of lymphocytes (immune cells) to recognize foreign allergens. The damage from light hitting the DNA in cells causes mutations, which years later result in changes that lead to skin cancer. This damage accumulates over the years. Photons (fundamental particles of light) hit the cells and structural fibers of the skin, generate destructive free radicals, and cause chemical changes in the cells. Sunlight also activates chemical "chainsaws" called enzymes, which cut apart the elastin and collagen structures that give the skin its stretchiness. The resultant skin is wrinkled, loose, and saggy, as you know from watching older folks who have spent too much time in the sun. Over-exposure also causes the skin to be irregular, with darker and lighter spots and scattered unattractive benign growths.

Controversy

The controversy over sunlight benefit versus danger rumbles on, with new data on both sides of the question. Clearly, early damage from excessive light exposure shows up later.

Several studies reported showed that exposure to two times the MED (the minimal amount of light necessary to cause redness of the skin) caused 100 times the amount of messenger RNA for collagenase, the enzyme that breaks down collagen in skin. Also, one-half the amount of sunlight necessary to cause redness increased the collagenase activity fourfold. Furthermore, even one-tenth the amount of sunlight exposure necessary to cause redness caused some increase in collagenase activity.

How do we make sense of such opposing information on the benefits and dangers of sun exposure? One way is to acknowledge that aging is a natural process and our challenge is to do it in the most graceful, healthy way possible. Living a full life exposes us to both those benefits and dangers; finding the right balance of sun exposure and using proper timing, shade structures, protective clothing, protective supplements, and topical antioxidants is the best we can do. Avoiding sunburn is most important.

Skin Cancer

Increased numbers of pre-cancers are abundant on the sun-exposed areas of light-skinned individuals as they age. Basal cell and squamous cell carcinomas appear to be related to sun damage, as do melanomas, especially in people with lighter skin. An additional risk factor appears to be the sunburn damage when a pale individual flies toward the equator for a one-week vacation, and wants to get a tan to show off that trip.

Studies have shown a 75 percent increased risk in melanoma in people who have had UV exposure from tanning booths, as well as an increased incidence of non-melanoma skin cancers. There may be other, yet unrecognized factors leading to the development of melanoma, but sun damage is definitely one of the known factors. One of the clearest indicators that sun damage causes melanoma was the experience in Australia, which was settled largely by pale-skinned people from the British Isles. Men worked outside in the warm weather without shirts, and developed a significant incidence of melanoma on sun-exposed parts of their body. Today, melanoma is considered a minor epidemic in Australia, and you can buy SPF 100 shirts there. Melanoma does have a genetic component; you are three times more likely to develop it if family members have it.

Sunscreens

Sunscreens definitely offer protection from sunburn, and some protection from wrinkling and formation of certain types of skin cancer. They do not protect against all types of damage, and there is some argument as to whether they may allow a person to stay in the sun longer, therefore increasing the chances of developing dangerous forms of skin cancer. One of the issues is the Sun Protective Factor (SPF) value given to sunscreens, which rates how well the sunscreen protects against ultraviolet B (UVB) rays. That means that if you're applying 15 SPF sunscreen 45 minutes before going out in the sun, you should have 1/15th of the damage and absorb 1/15th of the sun's rays that you would without it. Said another way, if you'd normally burn in 10 minutes, SPF 15 multiplies that by a factor of 15, meaning it might require as much as 150 minutes before you'd burn. The SPF on sunscreens is dependent upon applying a golf ball-sized portion of sunscreen to the skin, spread over the entire body. To make matters worse, applying less, such as half that amount, gives not half but a quarter of the protection, and so forth. So a little bit, as is usually applied, may give only a small fraction of the rated protection. Another confusing aspect of the SPF rating is that there is not as much difference as you might think between SPF 15 and, for instance, SPF 30. That's because SPF 30 doesn't give you twice the protection as SPF 15; SPF 15 filters out about 93 percent of UVB, and SPF 30 filters out 97 percent. So the difference is not as significant as it may appear from the number alone.

These numbers are based on Ultraviolet B absorption. More recently recognized is that ultraviolet A (UVA) rays also cause damage, including skin cancer and wrinkles. According to the Environmental Protection Agency, up to 90 percent of skin changes associated with aging are really caused by a lifetime's exposure to UVA rays. Many of the sunscreens on the market don't protect against UVA, especially ones from this country, and only now are we starting to import a few brands from Europe that do. You should look for sunscreens that give broad-spectrum or multi-spectrum protection for both UVB and UVA rays.

Another problem is that many of the active chemicals in sunscreens have estrogen-like hormonal effects. Applications of golf ball-sized doses daily over many summers may result in absorption of a significant amount of chemical to either activate the hormone receptors in tissues or disrupt the complex feedback interactions of estrogen and the many cells, tissues, and organs it signals. In the wrong situation, abnormal growth signals to target organs such as breasts and genitals can lead to premature development (look at how much earlier young girls are maturing) or to cancer growth. Add sunscreen effects together with other estrogen-like substances from plastics, pesticides, and foods and you increase its influence exponentially.

What sunlight does to the Skin

Let's discuss what happens when sun hits the skin. Packets of light energy known as "photons" hit chemical structures in your cells and activate them so that they transform chemically, which often causes them to combine with chemicals next to them. This includes causing chemical changes in the cells' DNA, which can eventually change cells into skin cancer. When you apply a sunscreen, the energy from the sun is absorbed by that sunscreen chemical, changed, and then released as a hopefully less harmful energy. Sometimes it comes out as a different wavelength of light. If the effects of that energy can be safely spread around and absorbed by the skin chemicals, there is little harm done.

Now think of it as if it were a football game. The football represents the packet of light energy from the sun. When the team hikes the ball, the opposing team attacks, the front line acts as a barrier, and the football is passed back and forth by the team in the rear to keep it from being attacked. The more the team behind the line passes the ball back and forth, the less likely a player with it will be attacked. We have a number of antioxidants in our skin, some naturally present, some from our diets (includes vitamin C, lipoic acid, glutathione, other bioflavonoids, carotenoids, and selenium), and some from substances we apply. If they are sufficient, balanced, and work well together like good linebackers, none of the team members will be attacked. Antioxidants not only help protect the skin (to a degree), they work together with other forms of protection, including sunscreens.

Some people prefer "non-chemical" sunscreens made with zinc or titanium. They absorb energy and give it off as well, similarly to other sunscreens. However, sunscreens with only these ingredients provide a lower SPF than those that include other chemicals. And the older, larger particle-size Zinc and titanium sunscreens leave a whitish coating on the skin that some people do not like. That problem was solved recently by breaking the particles up into very fine pieces, more similar to the size of the chemicals in the skin than the size of the cells. Unfortunately, there is mounting evidence that these tiny "nano-sized" particles actually penetrate the skin and may get into vital structures such as the nucleus of the cell where they can affect the DNA when hit by light. Because of this, I recommend that you use the larger-sized zinc and titanium sunscreens (check with the manufacturer to be sure what is in the product) and put up with the whitish color they leave when in use.

To make choices among the chemical sunscreens, use trial and error and know a little chemistry. Fortunately, you know a little more chemistry than you may have realized, just by knowing the English language. Get out your magnifier and look at the label on the box or bottle of sunscreen. If you see "cinnamate" or a similar word, you know that you do not want to use this if you are allergic to cinnamon or toothpastes containing cinnamates. Sunscreens that contain PABA or related chemicals are related to sulfonamides, so people who are sensitive to this class of medication should avoid them to avoid developing allergic reactions.

The protective effects of topical and oral antioxidants are discussed in other chapters. It appears that some antioxidants work by activating the cell's DNA to produce anti-oxidants. Small amounts of stress from gentle sun exposure may do this as well. Overwhelming the skin's capacity to deal with sun by producing redness or burning is not beneficial to the skin. Socioeconomic studies suggest that the people who go to the tropics for a short vacation and a quick sunburn so that they can come back with a tan are more likely to get melanoma than if they skipped these trips.

Sun Protective Clothing and Hats

My actual favorite barriers are sun-protective clothing. A number of companies make high SPF tightly woven synthetic fabrics that are lightweight and have vents built in under the arms, in front and in back. Pale people, including my wife, can enjoy vacations and activities in tropical climates while wearing these outfits, without concern about sunburn. I also find that wetsuit gear, from rash guards to lightweight wetsuit tops to full suits, protect well for swimming, snorkeling, and other water sports. Bathing caps and balaclavas made for swimmers and divers protect the head. All of these also provide additional comfort in cold water, protection from scrapes, and the safety of additional visibility to power boats.

Hats are another must for sun protection. They must be woven tightly enough to keep the sun's rays out (hold them up to the light and check). And they must have a wide enough brim, or cloth back and sides (desert safari style) to keep the sun off your entire face and neck. Baseball caps with a brim in the front do very little to protect your ears, neck, and the sides of your face. Wide-brim hats are now available from makers of sun-protection gear. Even with these, it may be necessary to use sunscreens, avoid peak sunshine hours, and take other precautions when you are near a reflective surface such as water, beach, white deck, or snow. This is especially true in tropical situations.

Summary

So what should you do about the sun, given all of this conflicting data about health benefits, accelerated skin aging, and possible skin cancer from sun exposure? I think this is a highly individual question, dependent on your degree of protective skin color, your family history and origin, your risk tolerance, and your priorities. If you are pale-skinned, blue-eyed, have a family history of melanoma or skin cancer, or burn easily in the sun, I think it is clear that you will look better longer and be likely to live longer without skin cancer if you are careful about limiting your sun exposure and protecting yourself from the sun. If you are darker-skinned, from the Mediterranean or similar area, and tan easily but do not burn, you may be able to safely tolerate more sun exposure over time. Still, you must choose whether you would rather look as tan as possible in your teens and 20s and therefore excessively aged in your 50s and 60s, or sacrifice the great tan to have healthier, vibrant skin for more of your lifespan. So, some suggestions to consider:

Avoid getting caught uncovered outside when clouds turn to sun, or allowing a brief stint outdoors to become an hour. Avoid show-off tans from one-week trips to the tropics that require initial burning and excessive time outside without protection. Do not depend on applied sunscreens for all of your sun protection—also use sun-protective clothing, sun shades, and careful timing of outside activities to protect yourself. Get the proper clothing and gear to protect you in whatever activities you enjoy outside. Remember that hazy sun through clouds can also cause sun damage and that reflected sunlight from water, sand, or other surfaces can be up to half as damaging as direct sunlight. Even light coming through a window, with most of the UVB-burning light removed, can add to the potential damage done by direct sunlight.

Once you have prepared to control your sun exposure, decide what kind of risks and tradeoffs are acceptable to you considering the possibility that you will live a long, healthy life. Consider getting 10 minutes of sun exposure on your body three times a week, or taking vitamin D orally to boost your levels of this important vitamin. When out in the sun, go inside to check your skin for redness, or use a timer to remind you how long you have been exposed. Above all, once you have taken protective measures and have made a choice about exposure, enjoy your time outdoors.

CHAPTER 11
A FUNCTIONAL PERSPECTIVE: FOOD, DIGESTION, AND THE SKIN

Let's imagine that you have a skin condition that is itchy, red, or swollen. It is likely that a biopsy of that skin would reveal an increased number of white cells around the structures in the involved area. We would call this immune system attack "inflammation," as we learned in Chapter 4, a word that indicates the heat and fire of the condition. White cells there are attacking something present in the structures or content of the skin. If you think about it, your next question might be "What are they attacking, and why?"

In some cases, the answer is that an infectious agent such as Staphylococcus aureus is causing the attack. Or it may be that, as in a disorder known as dermatitis herpetiformis, sensitivity to gluten stimulates an attack against the cells in an upper layer of the skin, leading to destruction of the cell attachments and formation of blisters. Sometimes the cause of inflammation is a chemical from a plant such as poison ivy or a preservative such as formaldehyde. In many other instances, the cause of the inflammation is unknown. Dermatology researchers may have found various body chemicals that are involved in specific skin disorders, but that is not much help in finding out what is triggering your particular skin condition. Indeed, most of the textbooks that I used during my training, in discussions of inflammatory skin conditions, listed the cause as unknown. When it is possible for dermatologists to find a cause by examination, history, or testing, they will try to eliminate that cause to control the condition. When the cause remains unknown and elimination is not an option, corticosteroids and other medications that suppress the immune system response or kill microorganisms are often used.

I found this answer of "cause unknown" to be unacceptable, and have devoted my life to finding better answers to that question of what is causing the skin condition. I had heard stories of skin conditions clearing when the patient eliminated certain foods from their diet. My research showed that cross-reactivity could be a cause for attack of one's own tissue stimulated by exposure to a particular microbial product or food. Expanding on what was known already, I began to suspect that other chemicals and food ingredients played a role in these inflammatory conditions. Following our discoveries regarding the nature of cross-reactive immune system attack in the late 1970s, I began searching for the *cause of stimulation* of a patient's inflammatory skin condition, two decades before these principles were published as common knowledge in the medical literature. As a result, I developed a deep understanding of the relationship between microorganisms, chemicals, foods, and skin inflammation. More than that, I was ready to accept teachings on food allergy, gut organisms, and digestion as scientifically founded, based on what I learned from my research. Accepting this premise helped me to understand the series of questions and answers required to translate this information into an ability to help people control their skin condition without the use of conventional immunosuppressant agents in the frequencies and doses used by my colleagues.

So the next question was to ask how a food could either get into the skin and cause a reaction, or could cause the immune system to react against this food and subsequently produce a skin condition. There had to be a number of different events to allow that to happen. First, tiny fragments characteristic of that food had to remain in the digestive system, and not be broken down completely by the digestive process. In chemical terms, this means that proteins could not be completely broken down into molecules of one, two, or three amino acids, but would have to remain in longer chains, known as peptides. To be molecular mimics, those peptides would have to be long enough to have similarities to unique peptides that naturally are present in the skin, even if they are part of completely unrelated structures. If they are in similar structures, there is even greater likelihood that these food-derived peptides could stimulate an inflammatory attack against the skin.

Those peptides would then have to penetrate the normal barrier in the intestinal tract, and enter into the circulation or the lymphatics. Some kind of defect would have to occur in the barrier for this to happen. We call this defect a leaky gut, a concept that is described in Chapter 6. There would have to be a reason why this leaky gut occurred, and possible reasons will also be discussed. Finally, these peptides would have to either escape any filtering in the circulation, or otherwise reach tissue in the immune system and create a response against them. How all this happens will be discussed in this chapter, as will the method to reverse this damage.

As discussed in Chapter 4, the immune system has several characteristic capabilities:

1. ability to attack very specific structures;

2. memory of the nature of those structures, so that similar foreign invaders can be attacked if they appear again;

3. residence of this memory in white blood cells both circulating in the blood, and residing locally in the skin where a previous reaction occurred;

4. ability to attack very similar structures to the original invaders they remember;

5. ability to carry out this attack on similar structures, even if the structures are part of your own skin.

We now know that there are both allergic reactions to foods by a variety of different immune system mechanisms, and pharmacological reactions to foods or their breakdown components. With that perspective, the way in which we search for the cause of disease changes entirely. Any exposure that seemed to precede the disease, or to change one's health, becomes suspect. Taking a person's medical history becomes much more complicated, because we cannot dismiss an infection, medication, or stomach ache after eating, simply because it was not listed as a cause of that disease. Observations must be refined to identify what could actually initiate the attack in the skin.

Foods and Functional Medicine

In the past, herbalists, naturopaths, nutritional physicians, and others used enzymes and other supplements to aid in various digestive processes (of course, conventional physicians did this as well, but only in more extreme well-defined conditions where digestive function was impaired). Herbs and supplements were also used to aid organs that are related to the digestive process, such as milk thistle for the liver. The broader understanding within non-Western systems of healing, such as Chinese and Ayruvedic medicines, substantiated entire systems of codification of relationships among organ systems in the body. This codification added new dimensions to previously perceived relationships among organs, supplements, and the treatment of disease. In many cases, early conditions could be completely reversed before actual "disease" became permanent.

The medical establishment often thought it was foolish to treat an organ that was not working properly but did not show up as "broken" or diseased on X-ray, physical exam, or routine laboratory test. If the liver was not enlarged on examination or X-ray, for instance, and the liver enzymes were "within normal limits," why not consider it normal and leave it alone?

It became clear that what was being done in the earnest alternative medical world was improving how organs behaved under challenge. It was not necessarily fixing broken organs, but improving how they functioned. The term "Functional Medicine," coined by Dr. Jeffrey Bland, emerged to describe treating to change the level of performance of organs and tissues under stress. Under that term, a vast number of treatments became codified into a coherent system that was consistent with and correlated nicely with observations in the medical literature. It put a new slant on interpreting the latest scientific research findings, and at the same time, moved many of the more solid "alternative" treatments with herbs and supplements into the twenty-first century.

Phases of Digestion and Ways They May be Interrupted

By weight, foods are the largest source of foreign material entering the body. In general, most people seem to handle eating without any problems, so we just assume that it all works fine. But when eating specific foods seems to trigger an individual's skin disease, we must reexamine the entire system to see where something went wrong. Foods have numerous ways in which they can affect the skin, immune system, hormones, and other aspects of the body physiology. Those effects depend on how the food is processed and absorbed by the body. If foods are not well broken-down by the digestive system, the remaining food particles are larger "molecules" which may contain chains of multiple amino acids; such molecules can serve as informational signals in the body or as stimulants to set the immune system on a course of immune attack leading to inflammation in the skin. With this concern in mind, let's take a functional medicine perspective in looking at the phases of digestion and a few examples of the ways they may be interrupted:

- **Cerebral:** The first phase of digestion occurs not in the mouth, but in the mind. We feel hunger, or we smell food cooking, and our body prepares for digestion. We may even find that our mouth begins to water when we are hungry and enter a store filled with delicious foods. This is the "cerebral" phase of digestion. Most religious and spiritual traditions recognize this phase with silence or a prayer of thanks before eating, bringing the mind away from the cares of the day and focusing on appreciation of the nourishing food about to be consumed. This important little pause offers a transition to a focus on digestion.

It is important to notice that our modern time-pressured world does not often allow such a redirection of focus. Little value is placed on time reserved for digestion. Digestion is a process that takes place best during relaxation known as "parasympathetic" activity. All phases of secretion of digestive enzymes, as well as the activity of each organ, proceed normally during this relaxed, parasympathetic state. Optimal digestive activity is halted during the fight or flight response of the nervous system's "sympathetic" activity to prepare all systems to confront or escape danger. If you eat while you are working, or bring the stresses of work home to the dinner table, you are likely to be restricting the release of digestive enzymes that break down your food. Although there are some cultures and occasions that cultivate relaxation, focus, and unfettered enjoyment of meals, it is safe to say that far more frequently there is a strong cultural pressure to remain mentally focused on work and keep the ongoing problem issues in mind, even while eating a meal; or worse yet, to simply grab a bite of food while still working. This is more than just a local issue. It is a cultural fault and a social disease.

- **Oral:** Chewing breaks food down into small enough particles for action of enzymes in the digestive tract to be effective. Enzymes in the mouth start the digestion of starches and proteins (which is why starches, such as bread, taste a little bit sweet when they are chewed for a long time). The amylase enzyme Ptyalin in the mouth converts starches to sugars. A lot of people today do not have the time or patience to chew their food well. Instead, they are encouraged by suggestions from the menu to "wash it down with a coke"—the same sweet taste as if the starches had been broken down into sugars, and readiness for the next bite, but not the same digestion.

- **Gastric:** Chewed food enters the stomach where hydrochloric acid, pepsin, and other digestive enzymes break down proteins further.

- **Intestinal:** When the acid mixed with food reaches the first part of the small intestine (the duodenum), the pancreas is stimulated to release a variety of digestive enzymes to break down the foods. The stronger the concentration of acid, the better will be the release of the alkaline pancreatic enzymes. These are the most important chemicals for breaking down the food proteins into amino acids that the body can use for building blocks. Incomplete breakdown results in chains of amino acids called peptides which are capable of cross-reacting with the body's own tissues and initiating chain reactions that lead to inflammation. Some of these peptides may also be signal molecules, which can then prompt other responses within the body.

There is more to the story. Normally, tight junctions in the cells of the intestines do not allow such peptides to be absorbed. Mucus secretions and specialized antibodies called immunoglobulin A (IgA) prevent the wrong substances from crossing the intestinal barrier and entering the lymphatics and blood-stream. Large collections of lymphoid tissue, called Peyer's patches, surround the small intestines and prevent entry of substances that might cause the immune system to over-respond in error. Modern antacids known as "pump inhibitors" also prevent the secretion of the mucoid secretions that protect the lining and integrity of the intestinal barrier.

• **Leaky Gut:** In a healthy person, food peptides do not penetrate the intestinal barrier. Functional medicine deals with what goes wrong and what to do about it. In functional medicine, the defect in the intestinal barrier that allows absorption of intact foreign material from the digestive system is known as "leaky gut." These foreign materials can be incompletely digested food molecules large enough to trigger an immune system response or send a signal to various organs. They can also be endotoxins produced by bacteria living in the large intestine that then enter the upstream small intestine (*see illustration page 147*).

When inflammation occurs in the small intestine, there tends to be disruption of the normal barrier so that larger food molecules that would normally be held within the intestines, can escape, usually between the cells of the inner layer of the barrier, into the surrounding capillaries and lymphatics. An overgrowth of yeast can trigger this inflammation and leakage. Following repeated escape through this barrier in the context of an inflamed gut immune system, the food particles from foods that are eaten repeatedly, too, begin to cause inflammation and further disruption of the intestinal barrier. As a result, some people with leaky gut build up a progressively longer list of foods to which they react, and a smaller and smaller list of foods that they can eat without a reaction. For them, this entire process has to be reversed.

Many foods contain lectins, which are proteins that bind blood group sugars on the surface of cells, allowing other substances to penetrate through cells such as the intestinal barrier epithelial cells. Beans and wheat gluten are examples of powerful lectin-containing foods that can initiate leaky gut and cause allergens to escape and cause further inflammation.

There are various other conditions under which the intestinal barrier is disrupted. Newborns, especially those who are premature or who have a family history of eczema, have poor barrier function for at least three, and sometime even 6 to 12 months. Any kind of reaction to foods or foreign material in the intestines that sets up a local response of inflammation will also disrupt the barrier. So an infant whose intestines react to cow's milk will absorb trouble-causing peptides of not only the milk, but of other foods eaten. This can be true of children and adults as well; in the worst case, a vicious cycle of reaction to everything eaten is created.

Labs that work with Functional Medicine can evaluate leaky gut by testing for the relative absorption of different material excreted in the urine. People who develop food allergy to whatever they are eating have clinical symptoms of leaky gut. If there is either clinical evidence of leaky gut, or the urine test is positive, elimination of specific foods and addition of dietary supplements can help. Many of the supplements for this problem contain glutamine, which functions as a kind of gut fuel. They also often contain various herbal substances, which help protect the membranes of the intestines with a mucoid coat.

Illustration
Gut permeability and leaky gut

What could be the source of all of those unexplained inflammatory reactions in your skin? Inflammation is often an allergic reaction related to the largest source of foreign material in the body: the food in the digestive tract, and the flora it feeds on. With normal digestion, that material should only enter the bloodstream in the form of amino acids and small peptides. But with poor digestion and leaky membranes on the border of the small intestine, larger peptides and toxins can escape into the bloodstream and the lymphatics, and act as targets for inflammation any place in the body or skin where those toxins are delivered.

Gut Permeability

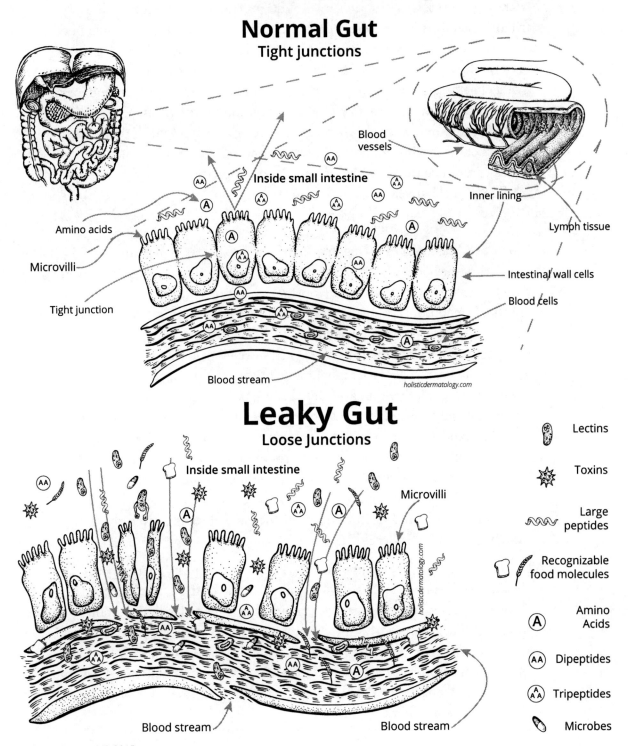

Normal Gut
Tight junctions

Inside small intestine

Blood vessels

Inner lining

Lymph tissue

Amino acids

Microvilli

Intestinal wall cells

Tight junction

Blood cells

Blood stream

holisticdermatology.com

Leaky Gut
Loose Junctions

Inside small intestine

Microvilli

holisticdermatology.com

Blood stream

Blood stream

Lectins

Toxins

Large peptides

Recognizable food molecules

(A) Amino Acids

(AA) Dipeptides

(A A A) Tripeptides

Microbes

© Alan M Dattner, MD 2015

147

- **The Large Intestine (Colon):** A large population of microorganisms, mostly bacterial and yeasts, live in the large intestine. There are between 30 and 100 trillion organisms in the digestive tract, and they interact with each other and with us. Some of these may be pathogenic and lead to disease. Some of these bacteria break down fiber in foods that our own digestive enzymes cannot digest. The organisms in our gut affect hormone metabolism, the tendency to be fat or slim, the tendency to have autoimmune reactions, and specific sites of autoimmune attack when certain bacteria are present. If pathogenic colon bacteria get into the small intestine and release their endotoxins, the toxins can escape into the bloodstream and lymphatics through a defective small intestinal barrier.

- **Probiotics, Yeast, and Intestinal Flora:** Infections (such as viral gastroenteritis) can disrupt the barrier. That is why limited bland foods, such as tea, are given until gastroenteritis is resolved and normal foods can be re-introduced. Other infections, inappropriate overgrowth of pathogenic (harmful) bacteria, parasites, and overgrowth of yeast such as Candida albicans, can also disrupt the intestinal barrier. Candida overgrowth is favored when antibiotic treatment destroys the normal bacterial inhabitants of the intestines, and allows other organisms residing there to take over the "parking spaces" once reserved for that normal population. Since Lactobacillus acidophilus, Bifidobacteria, and other "probiotics" contribute to the re-growth of normal intestinal flora, they are an important part of a program to restore the intestinal barrier. Studies have shown that probiotics restore tight junctions between cells, reduce the migration of organisms and large molecules across the intestinal boundary, and improve individuals with conditions such as leaky gut, as well as eczema (which involves food allergy).

This information remained in obscurity, known only among alternative practitioners and certain scientists, until recently when a relative miracle happened. Through scientific studies, major companies "discovered" special strains of probiotics that improved both the gut and the skin barrier. Somehow they managed to discover what had been known all along in smaller circles. The information began to be spread to dermatologists at major conferences such as the World Congress of Dermatology in 2007, where I heard it when I was presenting my own work.

What had not been officially discovered and presented at this meeting was the context, the surrounding factors, which contribute to and advance the positive effects of probiotics. Overgrowth of yeast in the digestive system, including Candida species, needs to be evaluated and treated in a more complete fashion beyond just probiotics, using a variety of additional treatments. Many of these treatments had been part of the practice of alternative physicians and practitioners since popular books on the subject had first appeared, starting with *The Missing Diagnosis* by C. Orian Truss, and William G. Crook's *The Yeast Connection,* and continuing with a flurry of popular books on the subject. Today, there are articles in medical journals on "prebiotics," substances that act as food for the probiotics to establish a foothold in the intestines.

Physicians tend to use potent anti-yeast drugs to kill yeast to try to solve the problem. Unfortunately, if they don't change the conditions that favor yeast overgrowth, the yeast comes back as soon as the anti-yeast drug is stopped. And what comes back are the progeny of the yeast that were most resistant to the drug. These drugs are important for serious yeast and fungal infections, and should be used in chronic situations only after conditions have been changed and the yeast population is as small as possible.

What conditions favor the yeast? Yeast grows on sugars and simple starches. Our population consumes 140 pounds of sugar per person per year, and large quantities of simple starches as well (white flour for example), that are quickly converted into sugar by the body. We should call our country not only "the home of the brave" but the "home of the yeast." The rest of the human population elsewhere in the world is doing a good job to keep up with us here in the US. Yeast issues are definitely on the rise.

Another dietary habit that allows the yeast to grow is lack of adequate fiber to keep the microbial population moving along. Use of antibiotics, steroid hormones, birth control pills, and other hormone preparations all favor the yeast. Less understood is the effect of eating other forms of yeast, molds, and their byproducts in preventing the body's immune system from throwing off the excessive yeast population in the gut. These organisms are all related, and they have a number of similarities in their surface "antigens." So the immune system sees many yeast and mold antigens when related products are eaten or breathed in (moldy houses), and judges them all to be "family." Technically, this is part of an immune system process named "high zone tolerance," part of the same process by which the immune system decides not to attack one's own cells in the body at the time of birth. Therefore, frequent eating of yeasty foods may inform the immune system to allow the yeast living in the intestinal tract to have a lot more parking spaces than it ought to have (*see Illustration page 153*).

• **Liver:** The liver filters the blood supply flowing away from the digestive tract. If foreign allergens and bacterial endotoxins have been leaking from the intestinal tract into the surrounding blood supply for a long time, you can be sure that the liver has been chronically challenged and overloaded. There are a number of herbs, nutritional supplements, and techniques that can support liver function and restore the liver's capability under stress.

From a functional perspective, one must evaluate and correct a whole sequence of steps to reduce an inflammatory process caused by ingested foods. These include:

1. Bringing the focus to appreciation and digestion before eating;

2. Eliminating specific allergenic foods;

3. Chewing food well;

4. Having adequate hydrochloric acid and digestive enzymes or supplementing with them;

5. Ridding excessive yeast, problem bacteria, and parasites from the digestive tract;

6. Taking probiotics to restore normal flora and gut barrier;

7. Eating adequate fiber and using herbs and supplements to reduce yeast before considering use of powerful drugs for this process;

8. Taking supplements to specifically support a better gut barrier;

9. Supporting liver function;

10. Eating a diet that supports a healthy gut flora that is low in sugar and simple carbohydrates, and high in various forms of vegetable fiber, so that it favors growth of beneficial bacteria in the colon and does not support excessive yeast or other pathogenic bacteria.

Any defects in function of the GI tract can expose one to gut allergens that lead to inflammatory diseases, including skin disorders. Correcting factors that predispose to inflammatory skin disorders can go far in clearing those skin conditions. Often, achieving optimal results is dependent on improving function in several organs.

ALAN M DATTNER, MD

Illustration
Immune "Tolerance"

How does your body decide what's part of you and what's not? Immune tolerance is the state of not reacting against specific targets, such as our own normal cells. Without immune tolerance, or when our tolerance breaks down, our immune system attacks our own tissues, as occurs in autoimmune conditions. In this first illustration, the immune system is tolerant to the proper populations of our own cells and normal resident microorganisms. Diet, antibiotics, hormones, and other factors can allow some types of organisms to increase greatly in population and the immune system will tolerate this. In the second frame, an overgrowth of yeast shows a harmful form of tolerance. In the third frame, steps were taken to reduce the yeast population by changing the ecology and we see a smaller, healthier population of microorganisms. In the last frame, dietary excesses (such as sugar or bread) show a regression, where the yeast population can grow once again, and the immune system tolerates the larger population.

Immune Tolerance

Specific immune non-respone to chemicals or organisms in the body.

Good tolerance

Immune tolerance is good, when you do not react against your own cells, body chemicals, or flora, and bad, when you do not react against tumors or infectious organisms.

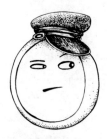

"There's a lot of you. You must be Self. I'll let you be."

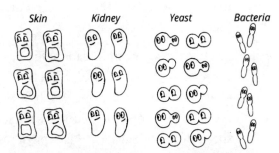

Bad tolerance

If conditions allow one type of organism to increase its population greatly over time, such as yeast in the gut, the gut immune system becomes more tolerant toward the yeast.

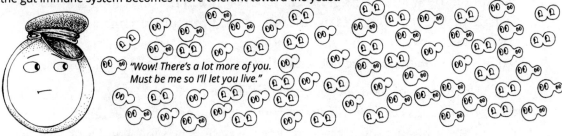

"Wow! There's a lot more of you. Must be me so I'll let you live."

Good tolerance

After a period of low sugar, low yeast diet, anti-yeast meds or supplements, and probiotics, the yeast population decreases and then immune system tolerance adjusts to a small yeast population. *holisticdermatology.com*

"Good to see a smaller, more normal population. I'll control you at this level."

Bad tolerance

But after eating a lot of sugar or a little yeast the tolerance is easily broken.

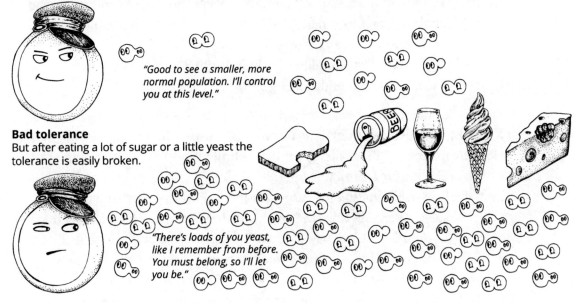

"There's loads of you yeast, like I remember from before. You must belong, so I'll let you be."

© Alan M Dattner, MD 2015

Food Allergy

Incredible as it sounds, the food we eat can actually cause a wide variety of different reactions in the skin and elsewhere in the body. Frequently people with one form of sensitivity reaction to a particular food also have different reactions to other foods. And they are often unaware that those reactions are related to their food.

These reactions can include rash, itch, and fatigue after eating, just to name a few symptoms. Some of the reactions are caused by a true allergic reaction, such as IgE antibody reaction, which is easily measured in the laboratory, and is also revealed by immediate redness on a scratch test. Only a small number of food sensitivities are detected by this type of testing, which is much better suited for immediate reactions such as inhalant allergies to dust and pollen. Varying testing formats each measure how other parts of the immune system can recognize foreign invaders. Each testing method identifies significant causes of reaction in some people, while missing them in others, and also can indicate a positive food reaction in some people even though no detectable clinical reaction has occurred (false positive).

Evaluation of food allergens starts with a trained ear hearing the patient's history. Symptoms beyond rash after eating, or eating certain foods; family history of food allergy, asthma, hay fever or eczema; occurrence following a history of yeast infections or conditions that might favor them such as repeated antibiotics, steroids, birth control medications, or pregnancy all are suggestive of food allergy. Aggravation by foods of the same plant families is also a warning. Primary tests for food allergy include IgE, IgG, intradermal, scratch test, and granulocyte (neutrophil, PolyMorphonuclear Leukocyte) enlargement, and antigen leukocyte antibody testing (ALCAT). Specific tests for gluten include antibodies to gluten, gliadin, and transglutaminase in the blood and stool.

Though these allergy tests are helpful, a careful history and food/reaction diary is really the best way to investigate what is causing the reactions. First and foremost, treatment for food allergy requires elimination of the offending food and its food relatives for a prolonged period of time. The gold standard for food allergy evaluation is eliminating the suspected food(s) for five days, and then reintroducing the suspected foods, one at a time, every three days, watching for reactions of any sort (if you have a tendency toward "anaphylactic reactions" with hives, swelling of the tongue and throat, and difficulty breathing, then challenge testing must be performed in a facility with an IV in place, an EpiPen® in hand, and airway assistance available). A reaction consisting of past symptoms may be immediate, or take two or more days to occur, depending on which of the different immune system reactions is taking place. Occasionally an individual's condition worsens initially, because withdrawal reactions occur for three days into the elimination diet; but such symptoms clear by day five.

Some people can tolerate traces of the food, such as the wheat in soy sauce, while others cannot. Taking digestive enzymes and supplements that help break down foods into their basic elements will aid digestion and allow leaky gut to repair. Removal of yeast, parasites, and unwanted bacteria also help repair leaky gut, as do supplements that coat the intestines and provide fuel for the intestinal cells.

The next mainstay in treatment is to eat foods on a rotation basis. Instead of eating the same food every day, eat it every three to five days, which provides a gap in exposure to the food and its potential allergens. With practice, planning and utilizing a rotation menu becomes much easier to do, and decreases the likelihood of becoming allergic to the foods in your diet.

Monitor your energy and symptoms for two days after eating suspected foods. A diary, reviewed with a knowledgeable doctor, including what you ate for the two days before an eruption, often has the key to identifying the cause of your problem. Remember that foods you crave, eat often, or to which you seem to be "addicted," are highly suspect. So are their "cousins" in the food family. Those cousins may be genetically related, as in different members of the broccoli family (Brassica), or biochemically and immunologically related, as in different compounds related to cinnamon, such as cinnamic aldehyde in toothpaste.

Remember that different tests measure different arms of the immune system, so that even if done properly, different tests may provide different results. Also, an individual may have several sensitivities in different organs of the body, giving completely disparate reactions to a series of foods. For this reason, it is important to record the list of symptoms that occur along with the food diary. Remember that symptoms can manifest up to two days after the offending food is eaten; therefore, it is important to accurately record what was eaten each day, to capture information regarding the entire two days that precede an outbreak.

Unfortunately, the allergy model does not tell the whole story of the effects of foods on the tendency to have allergic reactions. Some foods lead to a series of changes in the lining of the intestines, which causes inflammation, absorption of allergic intestinal substances, and finally reaction. Eating foods that aggravate yeast overgrowth may not cause an immediate reaction; instead, they may interfere with the intestinal barrier and make it easier for other allergens to leave the intestines and cause reactions. Think of eating such foods as "holding the door open" for other substances to escape the intestine and cause trouble elsewhere.

Some reactions to foods are not even allergies, according to the strict definition of an immune system reaction to a substance. Rather, foods may contain, or are broken down into, chemicals that are psychoactive and put you to sleep or confuse your thinking, as in the case of wheat gluten. Gluten may also cause a specific rash and injure the intestinal lining. A short chain of amino acids from a milk component, casein, has been called "caseomophine," because of its ability to cause sleep and other narcotic effects. More properly, these reactions are classified as food sensitivities, including both allergic and chemical reactions. Naming all of these different reactions as "food allergy" is often dismissed by conventional physicians, because some of these reactions do not meet the definition of true allergy.

Also confusing to many conventional physicians and patients alike is that the symptoms of food allergy may go beyond the typical allergic reactions involving itchiness, redness, swelling, runny nose, and watery eyes. In fact, symptoms can be felt anywhere in the body. Generalized symptoms such as sleepiness after meals, abdominal pains, bloating, skin rashes, and even repeated symptoms involving specific target organs are quite common. Different foods may trigger different reactions in the body. Skin may be only one area where reactions occur.

Taking away the offending food, such as milk, may be followed by a new sensitivity to the food, such as soy, used to replace it. Anything eaten repeatedly, day after day, can cause food sensitivity in susceptible people. One of the reasons for this is leaky gut as described earlier, when inflammation in the small intestines causes a breakdown of the normal barrier which keeps large molecules of incompletely digested food from leaking through the barrier into the lymphatics and circulation. Once they leak through, they can stimulate a reaction to themselves or *to other molecules that look similar to them*. Similar molecules may reside elsewhere in the body, for instance in the skin, brain, or other tissues; because of the potential for reactions to similar molecules throughout the body, the person affected may become sensitive to almost everything that seeps through the inflamed, leaky gut membrane.

Doctors who have studied food allergies have found that people tend to crave the foods to which they are allergic; in some cases, the body will block the allergic reactions triggered by the offending food., and that eating those foods could sometimes block the allergic reactions they set off. The body's effort to contain these reactions requires a number of compensations that may lead to bloating and lethargy. When the food is withdrawn, these compensations slowly leave, and the individual feels better in unexpected ways. Unfortunately, eating the offending foods again at this time may bring more severe symptoms than when the allergy was masked and compensated. Craving the allergic foods obviously makes it more difficult for people to eliminate those foods. As a result, people lacking will power, resolve, and a capability to control what they eat may have a very hard time with this approach.

Anti-Inflammatory Foods and Supplements

One of the key signaling systems of the body to manage inflammation consists of fat-derived molecules called prostaglandins (so named because they were originally discovered in the prostate gland). Prostaglandins have a variety of functions, including influencing pain signals and regulating inflammation. Some prostaglandins promote an inflammatory response. If these prostaglandins are induced, and you are in pain, you will probably take non-steroidal anti-inflammatory medicines (NSAIDs) and other Cox 2 inhibitors, which work by inhibiting the formation of these prostaglandins.

Other prostaglandins are anti-inflammatory. If you want to increase their numbers, you can do so with omega-3 fish oils. Our ancestors' ancient diet of local cold-water-grown foods and a lack of artificially hydrogenated foods, contained a much higher ratio of these omega-3 oils, and so did the bodies of people who ate that diet. This helped to reduce inflammation. People living in Northern climates today, eating hydrogenated oils, oils imported from the south, and meat or fish that are fed warm-weather grains rather than the cold climate plants, are more likely to have inflammatory oils which become inflammatory prostaglandins, and their blood tests demonstrate this. They have a tendency to have more inflammation, including dry, red, scaly skin conditions. Making a significant shift away from pro-inflammatory fats and toward consumption of omega-3 oils can contribute to calming some chronic inflammatory skin disorders.

Anti-inflammatory oils include omega-3 rich fish oils. It takes an informed consumer to identify the fish that are rich in these oils. For example, at this time, Pacific Salmon is a code name for wild salmon, rich in these oils, while Atlantic Salmon is a code name for farm-raised salmon that have been fed grains and food that are not rich in omega-3 fatty acids. Substitution of farm-raised fish in place of more expensive species is not uncommon, so that the consumer does not get the expected omega-3 fatty acids that are expected present in cold water fish. Cold-grown plants such as flax are also rich in omega-3 oils.

The proper shuttling of these oils into anti-inflammatory pathways in the body requires certain vitamins, minerals, and other factors. Foods can contain minerals, such as iodide, which supports the thyroid gland. On the other hand, unleavened bread products such as matzoh or chapattis, contain substances called phytates which bind out and remove minerals (including iodide) from the system, causing problems not only with glands such as thyroid, but other types of function in the body. Both changing the foods and adding supplements may be necessary to correct the mineral deficiencies that come from years of eating a deficient diet, or from a diet that stresses a particular enzyme system of the body, depleting the body's stores of specific minerals or vitamins.

Another issue with the food we eat and its relationship to our skin is pH balance. Our bodies must maintain a slightly alkaline pH to avoid inflammation. Everything we eat or drink affects our delicate pH. Simply stated, most animal products, sugars, and starches are more acidic and most green leafy plant foods are alkaline. We should all be eating in such a way as to increase the amount of alkaline foods we ingest and decrease the amount of acidic foods. Our convenience diet based on a few decorative vegetables, a large chunk of meat, and white flour desserts tends to push the pH balance of the body toward a more acid level. Without going into more detail at the level of controversy on acid base or mineral balance, it can be confidently stated that a diet consisting of a greater portion of raw and lightly steamed greens will shift the body pH toward a more normal alkaline level.

We should also be aware of how the chemicals found in pesticides affect our foods and therefore our skin. To have the abundance of food now available to us, we have freed ourselves from having to hand pick bugs off our crops via the extensive use of pesticides. Most of us were relieved when many pesticides, such as DDT, shown to be either toxic to the nervous system, carcinogenic, or otherwise dangerous, were banned in the U.S. However, these same substances were shipped to Central America and other countries from which we import our food. As a result, a large part of the population has been ingesting these fat-soluble pesticides for most of their lives, building them up in their fat cells. This is especially bad for those whose livers are not efficiently breaking down the toxic chemicals, who are overly sensitive, overly poisoned, or who do not have the genetic capability of eliminating the toxins. It can also be problematic for people who diet and lose weight, mobilizing pounds of fat in which pesticides and other toxic oil-soluble chemicals have been stored. Some toxic chemicals are bound to connective tissue, such tendons, joints, and the dermis (the tough layer) of the skin. Those chemicals which the body cannot rapidly expel are then redistributed into other organs, causing a variety of problems from headache to neurologic problems to allergy or even cancer. Directly and indirectly via the immune, hormonal, and liver function effects, these chemicals can lead to skin disorders.

Summary

Foods play a big role in causing inflammation that leads to skin disorders. Specific foods can act as triggers for an individual at a given time. When there are problems in the digestive system, the specific foods that a person reacts to may vary over time. One of the ways to control this inflammation is to identify and eliminate the foods that are acting as triggers. Additional ways to improve this inflammation involve improving all phases of digestion. Eliminating excess yeast and other organisms that interfere with the gut barrier or are predisposed to autoimmune conditions is also crucial for preventing exposure of the skin, body, and immune system, to allergens derived from foods and intestinal microbes. This chapter is an introduction to the various steps involved in reducing skin inflammation by working with diet and the digestive system.

CHAPTER 12
ALL ABOUT ACNE

Cindy's Story

Cindy had been a ballet dancer before she took on an office career. She always had a sweet tooth, which probably contributed to the gastrointestinal distress, acne, and slight weight gain was experiencing when she first consulted me. Another dermatologist had given her potent topical medications, which did not break the cycle of recurrent outbreaks in the middle of her menses. Her acne really broke out when she began having relationship issues last year. Cindy had tried a "cleanse" from a book she had read to clear the acne, but its only result was constipation. Colonics then cleared the constipation but not the acne.

I put her on a rather complete program custom-tailored to support her digestive system and liver; gave her supplements to help her hormonal balance; and got her to reduce her sugar intake, which helped in many ways, including being part of the treatment of her yeast issues from the long sugar habit.

In only one month she noted that her gas and bloating had diminished and her acne was improving, though she did have a small outbreak with her cycle. When she returned after the second month, having followed the diet and taken the supplements, she told me that she had not had an outbreak in the past month. Her digestion had improved, and her clothes were noticeably loose. It was the most improvement she had seen in seven months.

For many years, common knowledge held that acne is related to diet. In the 1970s, studies that were not well designed came out suggesting this is not so. Today, we're beginning to understand that there is a more complex explanation for acne; yet, it's difficult to discern the truth when so much misinformation exists.

This chapter will attempt to clear up some of this misinformation. Let's start with the basics: acne is the occurrence of inflamed or infected sebaceous glands in the skin characterized by red pimples on the face, prevalent chiefly among teenagers but experienced by many adults as well. Our understanding of acne has literally turned upside down in recent years. In the past, the accepted sequence of events was as follows:

- Plugging of a follicle;

- Increased twisting of the follicle, and other effects of hormones;

- Excessive or improper oil produced by the glands;

- Bacteria or other organisms growing in the opening;

- Enzymes from the acne bacteria breaking down fats to free fatty acids causing inflammation of the opening, causing blockage and deep destruction;

- Inflammation in the follicle.

The latest understanding is that inflammation in the follicle is the INITIAL event in acne. Most leading authorities still seem to believe that the *Corynebacterium acnes* (*C. acnes*) bacteria is the primary cause of that inflammation. I will explain here the factors they have overlooked.

Scientists have shown how oil, plugging, and inflammation are part of this process of acne, justifying the use of antibiotics to reduce bacteria, and retinoic acid to reduce cell stickiness, with proven benefits. But their explanation omits dozens of important factors, such as the nature of the oils in relation to diet, the blood chemicals secreted in sweat, the influence of food exposure on inflammation of the follicle, and the influence of nerve impulses on acne development. I will show how my experience identifies these factors as part of the generally unrecognized cause of acne.

Acne commonly shows up in the form of blackheads or whiteheads. Careful examination with a lens reveals that blackheads involve tiny "plugs" in the openings of hair follicles, consisting of dried oil gland secretion, known as sebum. The sebum gets "oxidized" in the air and turns black. These plugs can be removed by scrubbing with gritty soap, or by application of retinoic acid. They can also be extracted mechanically, by "acne surgery." This must be done correctly, because pressure rupturing the "sac" under the skin can lead to more inflammation and foreign body reaction. Bacteria introduced by fingernails or non-sterile instruments can cause infection; infection in the central face can go to the draining veins in the brain and cause death.

Prevention of infection includes refraining from constantly touching or "checking on" your face, even with clean fingers, and avoiding clothing and straps (such as sports head-gear) that rub on or touch the area. Use of gritty soaps can help, as can vitamin A creams and retinoic acid creams (by prescription from a physician).

The Application of Antibiotics for Acne

During my training in the 1970s, I was taught to use antibiotics such as tetracyclines to control acne. There were definitely some patients who were able to use tetracyclines for a relatively short length of time, taper off them, and remain relatively clear. But many patients, especially those with acne rosacea (a skin disorder in which the facial skin becomes oily, reddened and bumpy, and small red blood vessels are visible), seem to get worse when the tetracycline is tapered, and need to remain on them for long periods of time to accomplish control of their acne. One of my own long-term tetracycline-treated patients with rosacea, and several patients treated with long-term tetracycline by other dermatologists, came to me with intestinal yeast overgrowth issues and chronic fatigue syndrome resulting from antibiotic treatment. More recently, I have begun to see a number of patients whose acne worsened when their tetracycline was stopped. It seems the antibiotic killed off some of their normal intestinal bacteria, allowing an overgrowth of yeast in their intestinal tract, This assumption is unproven, but may account for why some of these patients benefit from probiotics. In these people, the benefit of the antibiotic on the bacteria in the follicle (described in the next paragraph) was negated by the effect it had on the intestinal flora. When the antibiotic was removed, the inflammation from the intestinal issues made the acne worse.

Oral and topical antibiotics are thought to work by inhibiting the *C. acnes* bacteria that live in the skin. Enzymes from *C. acnes* have been shown to break down fats in the follicle, forming free fatty acids, which have been demonstrated to cause inflammation. Current thinking is that this inflammation is what starts the process that leads to plugging and formation of acne lesions. Clearly this is a part of the issue, because use of oral and topical antibiotics, and even other antimicrobials such as benzoyl peroxide, reduces the number and size of the acne lesions. Unfortunately, they don't work for everyone. Additionally, in those patients for whom they do work, the use of the antimicrobial can result in selecting for organisms that are resistant to the antimicrobials; therefore, the antibiotics only work for a number of months.

The Evolution of Thinking about the Causes of Acne

As stated earlier, during the past 40 years, many dermatologists believed that the cause of acne was the plugging of the follicles, with the development of overgrowth of the *C. acnes* within those plugged follicles leading to inflammation. In more recent years, it is been shown that inflammation occurs as the primary defect, even before the occurrence of plugging. Current thinking focuses on the enzymatic action of *C. acnes* on the fats in the sebaceous glands and follicles. Hormonal aggravation from testosterone and other male hormone activity is considered to be an additional aggravator.

Some of the dermatologists whom I met during my training had come from an era before antibiotics were used for acne. They had direct experience regarding the effectiveness of dietary restrictions on treating acne. Before the development of antibiotics such as tetracycline in the 1950s, there were many more dermatologists than can be found today who spent time working with patients on what foods to avoid to avoid acne breakouts. Although some patients claim to experience an association between acne and consumption of foods other than milk and sugar, there is no clear proof of this association. This association bears further discussion as evidence emerges. Studies on the nature of sebum in the sebaceous glands have not yielded more than minimal clues as to what might be inducing the inflammation in acne. I look forward to someday bringing better data and clarity to this issue of food and acne.

Kevin's Milk Mustache

A young man named Kevin came to see me because the acne on his face was so bad that he felt uncomfortable being seen. Just *showing up* at school had become difficult. His schoolwork was suffering because he stayed home when the flare-up was bad. We spoke for a few minutes about his daily routines, the kinds of soap he used. He seemed to be emotionally healthy and stable, except for the embarrassment about his appearance. Kevin also mentioned that he had asthma and couldn't play basketball, his favorite sport, because it was too difficult to breathe.

I asked him about his diet. Nothing was out of the ordinary. And then I asked if he drank milk, and he casually said, "I guess." "How much?" I asked, and he replied, "I dunno, maybe half a gallon a day." Ah-ha, I had found my culprit. "It was Mr. Peacock, in the fridge, with the milk mustache!" I said, and he frowned at my reference to the board game Clue. I said, "Kevin, the bad part is that I'm going to ask you to eliminate one of your favorite foods: dairy. The good part is that we now have a pretty good idea what about what is causing your acne to be so bad. *And,* it's under your control." Kevin was understandably both dismayed and relieved at the same time.

When Kevin stopped drinking milk and started taking supplements for his digestion, his acne improved significantly. Furthermore, his asthma (which wasn't the reason he came to see me), also cleared up when he quit the dairy products. He had a double benefit from the elimination. I spoke with Kevin several months later. No longer embarrassed to show his face, he showed up at school every day. His grade point average had improved, and basketball was no longer a sideline industry. He joined the team and could play on the court without difficulty. On the phone, I could tell from his voice that the improvement in his appearance had also raised his confidence level.

One Size Doesn't Fit All

Clearly, not everyone who drinks milk has acne, and not everyone with acne will get better by eliminating milk. How you know whether milk products make a difference has both a difficult and simple answer. The simple answer is to stop milk products for a month, and see if acne gets better without it and worsens when you add milk back into the diet.

Many people think that lowering the fat content of the milk they drink will do the trick. However, three different studies have shown that skim milk consumption is associated with increased acne in three different populations. One of the primary authors on these papers, Dr. William Danby, has shown in a very elegant fashion how male hormone activity present in the milk could be a significant explanation of the cause of this milk-induced acne. The fact that this occurred in skim milk immediately reduces suspicion that the fats in the milk are the cause. Additional information that I learned in these articles supports my theory that the acne can result from milk-induced inflammation targeting the sebaceous glands: I learned that because skim milk looks very diluted compared to regular milk with fats, extra milk protein is added to give it a whiter appearance. Thus, another characteristic of skim milk is that it actually contains more milk protein than regular milk. So, there is a higher chance of having an actual sensitivity to the protein in the milk in the case of acne related to skim milk consumption.

Milk products are high on my avoidance list of acne triggers because of both the fats and the possible food allergies. Children in the United States are often given dairy products with every meal because milk contains many nutritional factors including protein, fats, water, vitamin D and calcium, to name a few. But for many children, eating the same foreign proteins day after day exhausts the immune system, and begins to create allergies that other systems in the body soon compensate for. The result is a hidden allergy, and various bodily mechanisms going awry, which eventually causes other problems.

For some, removing dairy from their diet seems really difficult (though it's becoming easier these days with all of the dairy substitutes on the market). These people need better proof that this is the culprit before undertaking such a hardship. It is here that careful attention to one's dietary and family history provides further important clues. Testing by blood test can provide further information to help make a decision. Analyzing all the information to determine whether or not a milk elimination diet alone will improve your acne, as you can see, is also difficult. It is even more difficult when you remember that it must be done while addressing other sources of unhealthy fats such as those in fried foods and large amounts of fatty meats.

Chocolate and Acne

Of course, milk is not the only edible that can cause acne. Armed with my suspicions, I administered an acne questionnaire to all my acne patients for nearly

18 years. That questionnaire had a section on diet frequency of several foods that have been mentioned in scientific literature as having a potential cause and effect relationship to acne. While my study was far from scientific, the impression was undeniably clear. Several foods, if consumed frequently, were very suspicious for having a direct correlation to acne—including chocolate.

Chocolate was one of the foods high on the list. Some women with acne craved it, especially around their menses. It has a number of biochemical and physiologic components that could be responsible for acne. These include sugar, saturated (milk) fats, paraffin wax in cheap chocolate that keeps it from melting (think of what that wax would do to harden the oils in your follicles and cause plugging), two major stimulants including a caffeine-like methyl xanthine known as theobromine and an amphetamine-like stimulant known as phenylethylamine. Food allergy to milk or components of chocolate and aggravation by stimulants are other reasons chocolate may aggravate acne.

Most well-trained dermatologists have been taught that chocolate does not cause acne. As residents, we read a study from our Harvard bibliography that showed that patients fed chocolate had the same amount of acne as patients who were fed a taste-alike treat that contained no chocolate. This very study has recently been shown to be flawed in its methods, and therefore wrong in its conclusion. An entire generation of dermatologists was trained in the false belief that chocolate had no effect on acne. And what about the other components in the taste-alike in that flawed study that gave it the rich, sweet tastes? Perhaps they are as important as the chocolate itself in causing acne.

I may be treading on sensitive scientific toes here, but give me a freight car full of chocolate bars and a high school, and I bet that I can change the "face" of that school. It must be emphasized that there are individual factors here, and that not everyone who has an occasional piece of chocolate will break out with acne. Chocolate seems to cause acne in some and not in others, which is why studies looking at a mass of people would show that there isn't a correlation. Chocolate has been reported to be a good source of anti-oxidants. Some people are more sensitive than others, and some women may be more sensitive at specific times of the month. Total volume of chocolate consumed may be the critical factor for some, while for others the total amount of sugar and/ or saturated fats or stimulants may be what is most important.

The Western Diet

Eskimos and Inuit Indians whose primary dietary component is fish from icy waters don't develop acne until they start eating a typical Western diet. This suggests that the omega-3 oil-rich diet they eat has protective effects against acne. Fortunately, this is one study that you can perform on yourself. If you have acne and feast on greasy foods, junk and fried food, etc., see what difference it makes to cut back. Dietary fats have long been suspects in acne occurrence. It seems both simplistic and obvious that a greasy diet leads to a greasy face. The kinds of oils that are absorbed from the food in the digestive tract and delivered to the oil glands in the skin are unquestionably related. Oils that have sustained a week at high temperatures in a fryolator have been oxidized and chemically transformed. So, too, have the meat fats been altered. All of these high temperature heated oils are high in Advanced Glycation End Products that combine and alter other body chemicals (discussed elsewhere in this book).

But we know that the chemical factories in the body do change the substances we eat, so how does this pertain? The oils that emerge from the oil glands have an important role in protecting the skin from drying out the way that old leather does. Leather is the skin of animals, and needs lubrication to remain soft; similarly, our oil glands help lubricate our skin and keep it from drying out.

Chain length of fats in the follicles can also be affected by the body's chemical factories. One of the ways that glucose (the sugar in the body) is stored is by building up the size of the fat molecules. Longer chain fats are termed "harder" because they tend to be solid rather than liquid at body temperature. We call this process of adding two carbon atoms to the backbone of the sugar molecule "chain elongation"; the longer the chain, the harder the fat, so eating lots of extra sugar and carbs can lead to harder fat. And the presence of harder fats in the oil glands is likely to lead to the plugging of the follicles that leads to acne. So the cheeseburger, coke, and ice cream dinner has at least two ways to aggravate acne just by thickening the oils your skin produces. Let's see how else these and other foods can cause trouble.

One good way to slow down flow at a tight intersection is to call in a battalion of police to investigate a crime going on. When you eat foods or chemicals to which your body is allergic, the white cells of your immune system think it's a crime. They come in squads by way of the interstate highway known as "blood stream" and on local back roads called "lymphatic channels." Once they become involved in investigating the activity in the follicle duct, they are seen as part of the white stuff, or pus, that fills the pimple. The swelling around the pimple is inflammation, which is designed to isolate and stop the "bad guy" chemicals, irritants, or bacteria. But in the wake of the immune system bringing out its big guns, bullets fly, and the swelling and inflammation that occur are part of the "collateral damage" that is done as the immune system attempts to gain control. So that big lump on your face with acne flare-ups might be inflammation caused by an over-reaction to something you ate.

Hormones and Acne

Numerous young women have come to see me for acne that got worse during "that time of the month." Many women's acne improved with diet changes plus a variety of supplements for the digestive tract, liver, and cleansing. There are several supplements that I have found to reduce outbreaks that arise during the hormonal cycle. One is a form of vitamin B-6, known as pyridoxal-5 phosphate. I suggest they take it daily, and then increase the dose right before the outbreak would be expected by the calendar. Many women have found this to work well. Be sure to check with your healthcare professional when taking high doses of vitamin B-6 daily for a long time because it can cause nerve damage. A rare side effect of B-6 is that it can cause the formation of cysts; however, most women can safely improve their peri-menstrual acne with vitamin B-6.

A number of hormones affect the follicle, most notably the male hormones known as androgens. Women who make excessive androgen in their ovaries often observe that their acne improves with birth control pills, which shut down their ovarian production of not only estrogens, but also of androgens produced by their ovaries.

Our environment contains a growing number of pseudo-estrogens. These are chemicals that turn on the same receptors on the cells as estrogens do, although they do so weakly. We have hardly begun to ask how a collection of these hormones will affect the follicles. Preservatives such as parabens, sunscreens, petrochemicals, pesticides, and even plant products (soy, for instance) contain pseudo-estrogens.

I lived in rural Connecticut for a number of years. My house was down the road from a dairy farm. One day on a visit to the farm, I was looking at the calves, and the farmer told me that 80 percent of the cows he milked were pregnant. I began to think of all the hormones pregnant cows produce. Those hormones are being released into their milk and getting absorbed by people who drink that milk.

Then I began to wonder if by chance those hormones might have something to do with the acne that milk-guzzling teens were experiencing.

Those pregnant cows have elevated levels of progesterone-like chorionic growth hormone in their blood, and in their milk. Some dermatologists hypothesize that these hormones may be absorbed from the milk. A good dose of hormonal content from pregnant cows would likely pre-dispose the oil gland structure to acne in some patients.

This is not the only hormone present in dairy cattle. Since 1993, dairy farmers have been using bovine growth hormone to make bigger cows with more milk production. We do not know how this may affect the follicle, and whether it may contribute to acne. It will be difficult to determine, because the FDA does not require labeling of milk to let consumers know whether this important hormone is in your "feed." The surest way to avoid BGH is to buy milk products whose labels state, "We don't give our cows BGH."

Another problem comes from the faulty breakdown and elimination of one's own spent hormones. The liver eliminates excess hormones by chemically converting them (in Phase I liver activity) and then coupling them in substances to transport them out of the body. When the liver is overwhelmed and not doing its job, it becomes difficult to remove not only hormones, but other follicle irritants from the bloodstream.

Estrogen refers to a whole class of different forms of this female hormone, some of which are beneficial, and some of which have been considered more harmful. Following diets that favor the conversion by the body of estrogens into the safer forms appears to improve acne, with the side effect of lowering the chances of developing breast cancer. Vegetables in the *Brassica* family promote conversion to the safer forms of estrogen. Brassica foods include broccoli, cauliflower, Brussels sprouts, kohlrabi, turnips, and mustard.

It also turns out that the large amounts of sugar we consume (estimated at up to an average of 140 pounds/person per year in the US), and the simple carbohydrates such as white flour which turn into sugar easily, have a strong indirect hormonal effect on acne. When a large amount of sugar is absorbed, insulin levels rise in response because insulin is needed to drive the sugar into the cells. When insulin levels become elevated repeatedly, the signal receivers on the outside of the cells, called insulin receptors, become less sensitive to the insulin, requiring higher insulin levels to effectively push sugar from the bloodstream into the cells. The high insulin levels cause the secretion of another hormone known as Insulin-like-

Growth Factor 1 (IGF-1), which appears to stimulate androgen formation and the production of fat in the oil glands in the skin. It works along with other hormones in men and women to aggravate conditions associated with acne.

There are a number of chemicals, most notably plastics, petrochemicals, pesticides, and topicals (such as sunscreens), that have weak estrogen-like activity. Although we often dismiss these compounds and their levels as being far too weak to cause effects in the body, it was recently shown that the level of bisphenol A (BPA) present in polycarbonate plastics has significant estrogenic effects. BPA also sneaks into our body when we touch the ink on the receipts printed by cash registers and other electronic printers. Phthalates present in polyvinyl chloride have also been shown to be an endocrine disrupter. And the plastic bottle substance usually thought to be safer, which is present in billions of bottles and food containers made each year, PET (polyethylene terephthalate), has also been shown to have significant hormonal activity. Yeast growth studies revealed that water stored in PET bottles had the equivalent of 18 nanograms per liter of 17 -estradiol. Additional studies showed that snails grown in PET plastic bottles produced more than twice the number of embryos as snails grown in glass bottles, further demonstrating the profound estrogenic effect of simply storing water in containers made of this material. Because so much of our liquids and foods have been and are stored in such plastics, it is no wonder that so many abnormal effects of hormonal influence, including acne and breast cancer, are being seen.

Topical Treatment

Topical treatment refers to applying substances on the skin and acne lesions. It usually does not cure the acne, but it does reduce the size and severity of lesions and in some cases can resolve them. Some of these treatments work by reducing the population of microbes in the skin, or by reducing plugging of the follicles. Some may even work by calming inflammation, and helping extract fluids and even toxic or inflammatory contributors to the acne lesions. It is important to remember that resistance can develop to anti-microbial compounds, so that treatment may work for several months, and then stop working because of the development of this resistance. Topical treatments make sense if the underlying cause of the acne is being addressed at the same time, to prevent new lesions from forming.

Since there is often involvement of microorganisms as a contributor to pustular acne lesions, antimicrobials can help suppress pimples. Some people find that natural essential oils dabbed onto the individual bumps, such as oregano oil or tea tree oil, are helpful for this purpose. These oils can be irritating if they are not diluted sufficiently and ineffective if they are diluted too much. Unfortunately, repeated use of essential oils can lead to allergic sensitivity, known as allergic contact dermatitis. This rash breaks out in a delayed manner, a day or two after contact with the oil, and may last as long as two to three weeks. People who are sensitive to fragrances (often containing essential oils) or who have other skin allergies, or just "sensitive skin," should avoid the use of essential oils for acne treatment. If you are one of those people and still choose to try applying essential oils, start with very dilute amounts (one to two percent) in a carrier oil such as almond, olive, or sesame, and slowly work up to higher concentrations, on just a few spots. Increase slowly, because the rash can take a few days to appear. When you have reached a concentration that helps calm down the pustules and does not cause outbreaks, you can begin to treat more than a few active lesions. Be aware that an allergic rash can still break out at any time.

Other anti-microbial herbs can be tried if essential oils seem risky for you. Beberine, present as a yellow compound in several herbs such as bearberry, Coptis, and goldenseal, can be applied as a tincture, spotted onto pustular lesions. Again, be sure that the tincture does not irritate or cause allergy, although it is much less likely to do so than essential oils. Only a drop of an alcohol-based commercial tincture is necessary, and should be spotted on only a few lesions. The biggest caution here is not to spill any on your white clothing or sheets, because it will leave a permanent stain. Immediate cleaning with rubbing alcohol may remove most of this stain, but care to avoid spills is best. One other caution, especially if you are into the club scene: beberine compounds fluoresce (light up) under ultra-violet lights, so if you are going to be in a place that has black lights, you may find that having your acne lesions light up fluorescent yellow is not quite what you intended.

Masks and other drawing compounds may be helpful for some. In the past, sulfur-containing masks were used, but they are not very popular because of the stench. Clay prepared as a thick paste can be helpful in reducing the swelling of individual lesions, and usually works best dabbed on at night. French green clay powder from the health food or beauty store can be mixed with aloe or witch hazel into a thick paste, and dabbed onto pimples and allowed to dry. Some people find that this reduces the size of lesion overnight. We have found that combining herbs and minerals with the clay enhances its healing effect.

Soaps can remove dirt and bacteria and oil from the skin. Those with very dry skin may find that soaps are too drying, especially in the winter, and will need to instead use plain water or cleansing lotions.

For those with a propensity for plugged pores and oily skin, gritty soaps may help to remove the plugs. Grit in the soap must not be sharp, or it can cut and irritate the skin, even if it is natural. Soaps containing salicylic acid may also help remove fine plugs and strip dead keratin from the skin.

Vitamin A products can also help remove plugging from the skin. They often cause a mild irritation, and should be used very carefully or not at all with other drying or irritating treatments, such as scrubs or fruit acid.

Conventional Topical Treatments

Prescription topical antibiotics can be helpful in reducing acne lesions, until the organisms involved become resistant. If these are dabbed on only to the few active lesions, rather than all over the face and back, they should not cause disturbance in someone who is relatively healthy. Since there is a theoretical possibility of development of resistance to the antibiotic used, I do not consider this a first choice treatment. Retinoic Acid products often cause lesions to worsen initially, but improve the situation after a few months. Benzoyl peroxide products can help to dry up acne lesions because of their antibacterial properties. If a patient has in the past has seen some improvement from such products and is still using them, I generally allow the use to continue, because my belief is that these products do not have much impact on overall underlying health factors. If you are progressing well with a natural approach but are not improving as much as you would like, then it makes sense to add some pharmacologic topical treatments to small areas. So I suggest you start by making dietary changes, then add natural topical treatments if needed. If that is still not working, then I would add conventional topical treatments.

Summary
Exploring Your Own Best Answer

Each patient is an individual, and I treat each according to his or her unique story. As you can see, each treatment has benefits and drawbacks, and holistic medicine takes it all into account. As with any form of healing, reactions are not entirely predictable, because of individual variation, and variations in the exposures, diet, supplements, and medications each individual is taking. I hope that hormonal testing and new tests in the future will identify those who respond well or adversely to both supplements and drugs. Until then, we must interpret each reaction to give us a better understanding of how each person's system works so that we can know how to treat. Recurrences of acne and adverse reactions should not simply be a stopping point, but rather an opportunity to explore the circumstances around them in to promote understanding more about the specifics of an individual's physiology and why their acne flares. Concentrating on bringing balance to the major disturbances, whether dietary, habitual, or hormonal, is a good first step in gaining control of acne. If the process seems overwhelming or does not bring the desired results, it is time to get help from someone experienced in the treatment of this disorder.

Science provides many answers, if one chooses carefully which scientific information to heed. A successful clinician takes the useful data, and combines it with her own life-long experience and her experience of the patient, in choosing the best therapy. Most, but not all, conventional dermatologists look at the studies on antibiotics and other pharmaceuticals for the treatment of acne, and dismiss the less rigorous information on foods. A popular misconception among the conservative branch of the medical communities, the ones who teach and regulate, is that if it isn't proven, it isn't so. That philosophy certainly eliminated a lot of useless bathwater over the years, but threw out many babies as well. As a result, diet was considered to be inconsequential or controversial at best in the control of acne by the majority of dermatologists and within the scientific medical literature for several recent decades. It is only in the past decade and the recent few years that the effects of high sugar/high glycemic diets, milk products, and probiotics have become recognized as affecting acne, have been recognized in the medical literature. The complexity of both diet and the way the body works are reasons that neither doctors nor patients easily grasp the concept that simple diet changes improve acne. Often a more complete understanding of the complexities is required for you to find the nutritional path to clear skin. This chapter should give you tools to initiate that path.

CHAPTER 13

DANDRUFF DOs AND DON'Ts: SEBORRHEIC DERMATITIS

Was it the white flakes cascading down your black sweater in the mirror as you prepared for a date, or your itchy scalp that prompted you to seek out this chapter? Maybe it was worse: maybe your condition failed to clear up with one therapy after another. Or maybe you are just curious. I am about to take you on a ride through the visions of my understanding, both scientific and intuitive, of the causes and treatment of Seborrheic Dermatitis, better known as dandruff. My goal is to give you more than just a prescription for treatment. I want you to understand the process that causes- dandruff, including some key points that are not part of the conventional medical understanding of the disorder or the marketing of anti-dandruff products. With this knowledge, you can work with your dermatologist and/or other health professional to achieve both superior care and results. The intent here is to enable you to have lasting relief from this problem as well as better overall health, rather than ongoing treatment with the potential for untoward side effects. As for my qualifications for writing this chapter, I have written the chapter on this condition in three editions of David Rakel's *Integrative Medicine*, and written guidelines for Integrative treatment of Seborrheic Dermatitis (SD) for the American Academy of Dermatology Task Force on Integrative Dermatology.

Definition, Description, and Diagnosis

Seborrheic dermatitis is the medical term for the condition that includes scaling of the scalp as well as redness and scale on the forehead, eyebrows, eyelids, facial creases (nasolabial), and other areas including the central chest. This is usually accompanied by a mild itch that may be annoying and is complicated by the reflex habit of scratching itchy areas and making them worse. The scale can be fine and dry, thick and sticking onto hair, or yellow and greasy.

Usually, physical examination and a history of when the condition gets better and worse is all that is necessary to make a diagnosis. A biopsy may be obtained if other conditions are suspected, but it is rarely a necessary step to confirm a diagnosis of seborrhea.

The scientific literature reveals an association between seborrhea and a particular genus of yeast that lives in the hair follicle, previously called *Pityrosporum* and now called *Malassezia*. Some studies have shown that there are more *Malassezia* species in the skin in people with seborrhea than in normal people without seborrhea, but other studies do not report this. It is only in the context of the possibility of an *increased inflammatory reaction* to those *Malassezia* species that one can understand the relationship of the yeast to the seborrhea: both the yeast in the follicle and an allergy to that yeast are needed to produce seborrhea.

There are plenty of anecdotal reports suggesting that there is some connection between the nervous system and seborrhea. The best-known connection is an aggravation of the condition in response to anxiety. There are also reports of cases of seborrhea breaking out at the site where an injury to the nerve causes a loss of sensation. There are even reports of seborrhea occurring with an onset of the neurodegenerative disease, Parkinsonism.

Another instance in which severe seborrhea occurs is in persons with HIV/ AIDS. It seems to be associated with an overgrowth of the *Malassezia* yeast, as well as specific changes in the immune system related to the disease.

What Is It Related To? What Else Might It Be?

Fungus can cause a scaly rash on the skin (not often on the face), usually with redness and a raised scaly border. Sometimes fungal scraping and even a culture are necessary to be certain that the condition is not caused by a fungus. Ringworm of the scalp can also cause scale, but the pattern is more often round, with more hair loss inside the circle. There are many other causes of scaling and redness of the skin. Eczema, or atopic dermatitis, is the most common (see chapter 14). Some physicians feel that eczema is related to seborrhea; others believe that patients with seborrhea may have allergies and allergic tendencies.

If the scaling on your scalp and elsewhere is very thick, your condition might actually be psoriasis (see chapter 16). There seems to be some relationship between seborrhea and psoriasis, and in some cases the distinction between the two is difficult to make at first glance. Indeed, there is a kind of crossover condition with thick scale in the scalp known as sebo-psoriasis.

This chapter can help you begin to understand the underlying causes and routes of treatment of seborrhea. It is not a complete self-diagnosis guide, at least in part because it is impossible to know what else might be occurring in terms of both this condition and your overall health. If you have a problem with dandruff, your dermatologist should evaluate your condition. You can then use the information contained in this chapter to inform you about some of the steps (in addition to the care prescribed by your physician) that you can take to control this condition long-term.

Background on Yeast and Seborrhea

Let's look back a few decades to appreciate how our understanding of this condition has evolved. My first chief of dermatology, Dr. Frank Pass, told me the following story. A chemist was given the job of developing a shampoo to combat dandruff. Cleverly, he observed that there was a type of yeast in the follicles in dandruff, so he developed a shampoo directed against the yeast. It worked, and that was the origin of zinc pyrithione shampoo, which became widely used in anti-dandruff shampoos such as Head and Shoulders.

What has been puzzling is that, although studies show the presence of *Malassezia* or even the increase of *Malassezia* in the follicles associated with seborrhea, other studies show that the abundance of *Malassezia* alone is not sufficient to determine whether or not Seborrhea will occur. This suggests that some other important factor is involved. More recently, specific strains of *Malassezia globosa* and *Malassezia restricta* have been linked with seborrhea. Furthermore, it has been demonstrated that these two strains produce a lipase (an enzyme that breaks fats down to free fatty acids) that appears to irritate the follicle and lead to the scaling. Additionally, oleic acid has been identified as a cause of scaling, even independent of the *Malassezia*.

Malassezia yeast is dependent on the lipids in the skin. Studies show that yeast in the follicles release enzymes that cause scaling by breaking down fats to free fatty acids, leading to irritation, inflammation, and subsequent scaling.

There still seems to be an unexplained inflammatory reaction that may not be based on free fatty acid inflammation alone. Medical researchers were looking for a standard, more simplified formula. One disease, one cause. More of the cause should give more disease.

My Big Ah Ha! and Shift in Thinking

When I worked in the NIH laboratory in the late 1970s, our research results caused an incredible shift in thinking for me, and new insight into what occurs when people get seborrhea. This insight was one that neither the pharmaceutical industry nor my colleagues seemed to have recognized. In the lab, we found that exposure of cells from the immune system to one foreign material could cause a reaction to a related but different material. Therefore one type of yeast initiating an immune system response could cause a reaction *to another, similar, type of yeast elsewhere in the body.*

My big "ah ha!" was that it was not just the presence of yeast in the follicle, but the *reaction against* yeast in the follicle that was the key to dandruff! This suggested that other types of yeast in the body could be the very trigger to initiate this response. **In other words, seborrhea appears to be caused by intestinal dietary yeast allergens inciting a reaction that causes an immune system attack against the yeast in the skin hair follicles, leading to redness and scaling in people predisposed to this specific reaction.**

So what might be the source of this other yeast? First, an overgrowth of yeast in the gastrointestinal tract is a problem that alternative medicine acknowledges more fully than conventional medicine does. We also know that items among our food supply, such as bread, wine, beer, and fermented foods, are full of yeast and yeast byproducts, and these could also initiate an immune system reaction against yeast in the skin follicles. So we don't have a single cause, but rather a whodunit with an instigator and a victim, *both* of which are required to trigger an outburst against a target in the follicle.

The best news of all is that these probable causes can be identified, and with some difficulty but little danger, be eliminated from the diet. And we can use this thinking to predict other exposures that might contribute to causing the disease. An even more radical notion is that this awareness not only places responsibility for the problem, but also the solution to the condition, directly in the hands of the person suffering from dandruff.

Do you see what an advance in understanding can do to shift the perspective about the care of a disorder? Let's review it because it is so crucial to fully understand the process. It's not only the microorganisms (the yeast and bacteria) that cause an inflammation, but also their *resemblance* to some other existing target of the immune system, being attacked elsewhere in the body. The target could be another microorganism, the structures that microorganisms inhabit, or a specific tissue, cell, or molecule. Any of these may provoke a response, causing the body to "kick up a fuss." Like road rage, the fracas is caused not by the actions of only one driver, but also by the degree of reaction from the second driver.

Now let's look at two other details of this equation. We know from my own research as well as from many studies in the medical literature that when the body's defense system recognizes the tiny characteristic fragments of these organisms, it responds with a reaction. We call these tiny fragments "antigens." They often consist of a chain of protein building blocks called amino acids. You can picture this chain as linked miniature sausages. The body's defense system recognizes this "sausage chain" also when it is presented in a kind of "bun." The "bun" (the part of self that is recognized) is your transplantation antigen (the aspect that needs to be matched to accept a transplanted organ). The immune system recognizes the whole object (the sausage chain and bun combined). So it is a little of you and a little of the foreign matter in question that is recognized as a whole sandwich. Any alterations in the bun or the sausage chain may change the recognition (so hold the mustard).

Let's discuss a completely different example to illustrate the likely process taking place. Imagine that you are introduced to someone at the beach who is wearing casual beach clothing. Some days later, you meet him all dressed up in a suit, and for a few moments, you can't actually recognize him. What is happening is that you recognize the individual not just as a face or a body, but also in the context of a particular outfit and location. That is exactly how the cells of the immune system recognize the pieces of foreign material, secretions, and toxins of the yeast. And that context is a unique structure of the person's own individual genetic makeup: their transplantation antigens (known as their Major Histocompatibility Complex or MHC). In the same way that a matching blood type is required for a safe, non-reactive blood transfusion, matching transplantation antigens are required for a body to receive an organ such as a kidney without rejecting it. Like the beach, bathing suit, and body, the transplantation antigens provide the context for recognizing the foreign antigen or "face" of the invader. Not only is it difficult to recognize a person who we see out of context, but we can also easily confuse someone we met briefly at the beach with someone we met elsewhere who looks similar to the one at the beach. Our body's immune system cells, the lymphocytes, can sometimes make the same mistake.

What that means in regard to seborrhea is that though the lymphocytes go into battle to fight off intestinal yeast allergens, when they encounter yeast in the hair follicles, they think it's the same "enemy" and begin to attack there as well, causing the redness and scaling we see as seborrhea (*see Illustration next page*).

Illustration
Seborrhea (Dandruff)

What causes dandruff? Excess Candida (and other related yeast and yeast by-products) in the intestinal tract and surrounding lymphatics is recognized by the immune system as bad guys and is attacked by T-lymphocytes. These lymphocytes then divide and produce more lymphocytes that recognize and attack the yeast in the gut. When those new, sensitized lymphocytes circulate and reach the hair follicle apparatus in the skin, they recognize the local (Malassezia) yeast because it is similar to the Candida. So they attack the Malassezia yeast, too, and this inflammatory process triggers a rapid cell division of the upper layer of the skin, leading to redness and scaling.

Seborrhea-Dandruff

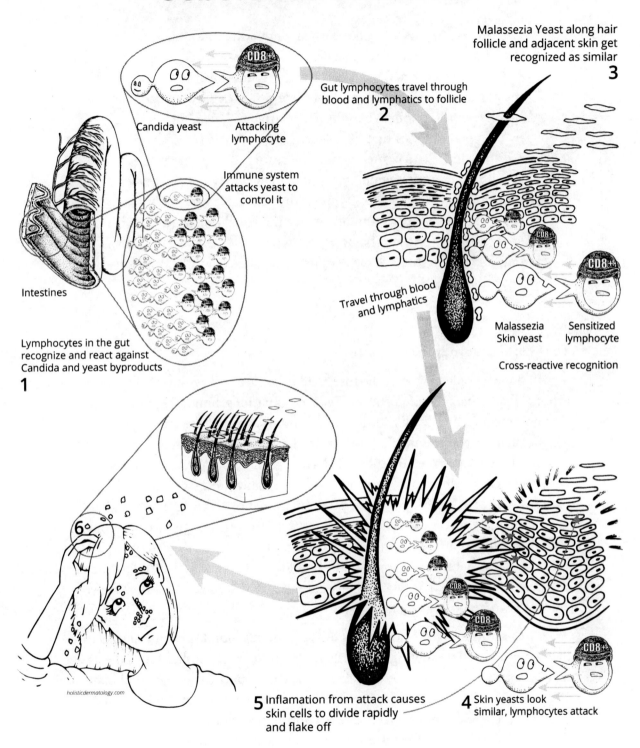

Malassezia Yeast along hair follicle and adjacent skin get recognized as similar
3

Gut lymphocytes travel through blood and lymphatics to follicle
2

Candida yeast   Attacking lymphocyte

Immune system attacks yeast to control it

Intestines

Travel through blood and lymphatics

Malassezia Skin yeast   Sensitized lymphocyte

Cross-reactive recognition

Lymphocytes in the gut recognize and react against Candida and yeast byproducts
1

6

5 Inflamation from attack causes skin cells to divide rapidly and flake off

4 Skin yeasts look similar, lymphocytes attack

holisticdermatology.com

© Alan M Dattner, MD 2015

The Candida Connection

Candida is the most common yeast living in the intestinal tract. It is normal if it restricts itself to a limited number of "parking spaces" in your digestive tract, but when it starts to take over too many of the parking spaces, it becomes a problem for the healthy bacteria that live in the colon. When those bacteria are killed, for instance by taking antibiotics that kill bacteria but not yeast, the Candida cells reproduce and confiscate more territory. They feed on simple starches and sugars, which are unfortunately, an ever-increasing portion of the human diet in our culture. So our dietary habits are supporting a culture of Candida in our intestinal tracts. And this is an aggravator for Candida overgrowth, which then can cause our immune system to attack the yeast in our skin, causing inflammation and seborrhea: this is clearly a case of "culture shock."

The Short Fuse Syndrome

Some people have a "short fuse" and become angry with very little provocation, while others remain calm in the same situations. Similarly, some people's skin becomes red and scaly with little provocation. One of the reasons for this is an information communication system in the body that is based on oils. More specifically, it is based on particular oil-derived signal molecules that are known as "prostaglandins," which play a role in regulating many processes, such as opening blood vessels or increasing or decreasing inflammation. The term prostaglandin came from early observations that secretions from the prostate gland could control physiologic functions. So the unseen substances were named "prosta-gland-ins." We now know that they are composed of building blocks of fat called fatty acids. Furthermore, these fatty acids are "unsaturated," which means that they are very vulnerable to becoming rancid.

Unsaturated fatty acids have at least one double bond (a chemical structure that is more reactive) waiting anxiously to combine with another molecule; they will become either saturated, oxidized (rancid), or part of a new combination structure. These unsaturated fats must be protected with anti-oxidants such as vitamin E. These are most effective when your body isn't under oxidative stress. Oxidative stress occurs, for instance, when you exercise while not in condition, when you eat foods that have been fried at high temperatures, or when you subject yourself to excessive sun exposure. So if you're experiencing a tremendous amount of oxidative stress, you might want to wait until you've gotten that under control before you take your unsaturated omega-3 oils.

One of the painful constraints of scientific medicine is that it restricts us from making statements until the facts are absolutely proven. I say painful, while thinking about the millions of smokers who lost good years of their lives or suffered in other ways from a habit that, until recently, lacked scientific proof that it was harmful. We were unable to make such claims on the basis of what appeared to be happening, or what seemed to make sense when you saw the burning smoke going into a person's lungs, and lungs turning black after a lifetime of smoking. Viewing the situation holistically, formal studies are not required to conjecture that smoking is harmful.

Similarly, one can wonder what happens to all the poor quality and harmful fats and fat-soluble chemicals that enter a person's body on a regular basis. These include high temperature heated oils from frying, baking, and grilling, loaded with advanced glycation end products; fat-soluble pesticide residues in foods; preservatives; toxins from packaging plastics; and chlorinated compounds such as PCBs. One has to hope that they don't become part of or alter the building blocks of that most critically important organ, consisting mostly of fat-related substances, that sits on top of your spinal cord. Of course I am referring to your brain, which is crucial to your survival and enjoyment of life. I would even venture a wild guess that the oil glands in the skin (sebaceous glands) might have a role in secreting these harmful oils and fats to expel them from the body. So people with the oily form of seborrhea (sebo = oil, rhea = rapid flow, as in diarrhea) might be dumping unwanted oils through the skin. If this is the case, then seborrhea is a protective process, and it would make good sense to eliminate the oils on one's head and in one's diet as well.

Effects of the Type of Oils Consumed and Seborrhea

This brings up the subject of oils in one's diet. The first priority is to get rid of bad oils. Let me discuss what I see as bad oils and why I view them as harmful, so that you can evaluate your diet in light of changing opinions about good and harmful fats. Examples of potentially harmful oils include:

• Oils that have been heated to high temperatures in the process of frying or are hydrogenated to retard spoilage. These may have trans-saturated fatty acids, which cause a number of problems that I will discuss later.

- Oils that are rancid are just as bad for us. These often give the bitter aftertaste you may remember from eating nuts that sat around too long.

- Oils that come from plants sprayed with DDT and other pesticides carry these neurotoxins into your brain. Petroleum derivatives related to auto and other industries are not good building blocks for human tissues.

- Oils that have toxic or carcinogenic properties, such as cutting oils.

Based on this premise, we would expect the skin, if it were a good team player for the rest of the body, to dump these bad oils and toxic substances and the nearby skin containing them, as fast as it could. The process would have the appearance of oily skin with ample scale being shed. In other words, its appearance would be similar to that of seborrhea!

If this is a problem triggered by bad oils, then which oils are good or even helpful? Mono-saturated plant oils with a long history of use (for example, olive oil) are good oils for consumption. In general, plant seed oils tend to be acceptable as well; however, the way in which they have been squeezed, processed, and stored makes a substantial difference in their freshness and acceptability. The oil should be cold pressed, packed in liquid nitrogen, and should be stored cold in the refrigerator.

There are also some oils that actually can help eliminate bad dandruff. These oils are able to calm the tendency toward inflammation. The most important of this group is omega-3 unsaturated fatty acid. The most active oil in this class is fish oil, and specifically the eicosapentaenoic acid (EPA) component of fish oil. Flaxseed oil, containing alpha linolenic acid, is another important oil in this class, but it requires a number of transformations in the body to work as an anti-inflammatory agent. Not everyone's body can efficiently perform those steps, so its effectiveness varies from person to person.

Of course, it is equally important to drastically reduce or eliminate oils containing trans saturated fatty acids. Fortunately, many such products are now widely available and advertised as free of these harmful fats. Unfortunately, many products sold in convenience stores maintain their long shelf life because of these oils, and partially hydrogenated oils still appear on the labels of many prepared foods. This means that you must read labels carefully. Fried foods contain these oils because they are formed during the process of frying.

So far, I have discussed the oils in foods that lead to either increased or decreased inflammation. You've probably guessed that most of these oils need to be converted in our body to the chemicals that signal our system about how to behave. Those conversions require chemical machines in the body known as enzymes, and each of those enzymes requires a supporting team of other vitamins and minerals known as cofactors. Just as a racecar cannot win without a good pit crew, the right fats cannot give you the best result without the support of other team components. Some of the necessary components for the enzymes to keep the oils anti-inflammatory include vitamin C, vitamin B-complex members, zinc, and magnesium.

Scale of Severity

At the low end of the scale of severity is occasional flaking of the scalp with no redness or itchiness, which doesn't cause any embarrassment and goes away with shampoo. As the scaling of the flakes gets thicker, more persistent, more widespread, and harder to remove, severity increases. Redness on the scalp, face, and forehead also causes more concern for both appearance and possible underlying issues, as does itching. When all these symptoms appear and the body is impacted as well, patients need more help than medicated shampoos can offer.

I gain much information from just listening to my patients. When their diets contain many problem fats and oils and many sugar- and yeast-laden foods, or if treatment with antibiotics preceded the symptoms becoming worse, I suspect these food items as significant contributing factors. If there are other allergies, I explore their contributions as well.

Treatment: Anti-yeast Program

The basic anti-yeast program has two primary aspects. First, stop feeding the yeasts that live in your digestive tract by substantially reducing sugars and simple starches in your diet.

The second aspect of this dietary plan is to stop eating foods that are made of yeast, yeast byproducts, and also their cousins, molds and fungi. Suggestions for how strict to be about this elimination vary in different yeast books because some people are much more sensitive than others, and the sensitivity actually increases in the early stages of the elimination diet. It's as if your immune system has many antennae looking for yeast. When you remove most of the yeast, there are more empty antennae with their feelers out looking for yeast, so even a little bit sends them into high alert. Gradually, if yeast exposure is limited for long enough, the immune system drops many of its yeast antennae because they have been sitting around without work for such a long time.

Changing the balance of essential fatty acids (EFAs) in the body is a key to controlling seborrhea. Notice that I said changing the balance, rather than taking supplements of EFAs. That's because it's important to reduce the intake of harmful fats and at the same time increase the intake of helpful ones. A layer known as a membrane surrounds each cell in our body. This "membrane" is made up of a double layer of fatty acids, which are the breakdown products of fats and oils that we eat. Some of these fatty acids are snipped off and made into messengers, to be used when the cells want to send signals. Which oil the membrane consists of will determine whether the signal will call for calming or for inflammation. Trans-fats, saturated fats, and other common fats in our diet lead to signals that tend to generate inflammation. Omega-3 fats and some omega-6 oils result in less inflammation.

My first recommendation is to follow the "Mediterranean diet," which will help you avoid the trans-saturated fats that are important for long shelf life in prepared foods: eat fresh vegetables, and consume as few prepared foods as possible. Olive oil is traditionally recommended, because of the benefits of the oleic acid it contains, but some recent studies suggest that safflower oil may be as good or better. Recent reports reveal that patients sensitive to seborrheic dermatitis, but not non-sensitive individuals, develop scaling when oleic acid is applied to their scalps. So some people may benefit more from Safflower oil, rich in linoleic acid (which is different from the oleic acid of olive oil), used for salad dressings and non-heated food preparation.

Eating cold-water fish will put omega-3 fats directly into your diet. You can also use omega-3 enriched fish oil. Its two ingredients are the anti-inflammatory EPA, and then DHA. It is important that the oils have been purified to remove both mercury and PCBs. They should either be packed appropriately to prevent spoilage (brown bottle, nitrogen sealed in to eliminate oxygen) and/or be shipped cold. These oils will spoil if left in the sunlight or exposed to the air, or if you don't refrigerate them after opening.

If you are a strict vegetarian, flaxseed oil is a good source of omega-3s, but, as stated earlier, they are in a different form that has to be converted by the body to be useful. The carbon backbone that makes up the molecule is 18 rather than 20 carbons long, and has to be elongated in the body to provide its full anti-inflammatory effect. Because not everyone's body can perform that process efficiently, some people will not benefit as much as others from the flaxseed oil.

There are other oils of a different class, known as omega-6 unsaturated fatty acids, which also reduce inflammation. These are found in evening primrose oil, and in even greater concentration in borage oil. Incorporating these oils into your diet can also help reduce inflammation.

Joe's Story

A patient of mine named Joe always tried to look his best, especially by the way he dressed; but he had a slightly unkempt air about him. The most definable aspect of that air was the red scaly rash prominent on and between his eyebrows, around the corners of his nose, and across his forehead below his hairline. Having just a touch of edginess in his demeanor didn't help. The rash really made it uncomfortable for him with his work in sales, and the flakes on his clothing made it impossible for him to wear a dark suit. Because he enjoyed outdoor exercise, his sweet tooth did not make him overweight. He enjoyed a beer after work on a regular basis, and sandwiches and pizza were a staple in his busy work routine.

I explained to him the relationship between the yeast he was growing in his gut and all his sweets and simple carbs, plus all the yeast and fungal products in the bread, cheese, and beer he was consuming. He wasn't too happy at first with the idea of giving up some of his favorite foods, but he was really motivated to present a good appearance for his sales work. Shampoos he had tried so far had only given him temporary relief; he knew from a shiny spot (from steroid atrophy) that was beginning to appear near his hairline that he could not tolerate the repeated use of topical steroids any longer, which also provided only temporary relief anyway. So he decided to follow the diet and the anti-yeast regimen. This, along with omega-3 oil supplementation and the occasional use of an anti-dandruff shampoo, made a big improvement in his seborrheic dermatitis rash, and was enough motivation to keep him on the diet. Occasionally he slipped on the diet, and the redness and scaling come back.

Ridding bread from the diet eliminates wheat as well as yeast, and wheat is one of the most common food allergens. Making any of these changes certainly will eliminate some commonly-eaten foods, and those foods just may be the ones that are causing trouble.

I once saw a patient with seborrhea and neuropathy who improved on large doses of various B vitamins. You may have guessed that if there is a connection between conditions of the nerves and seborrhea, then there is probably some connection between that great big nerve control bionic computer on your shoulders that is taking all this in, and what happens on your scalp. It's interesting to note that some people who feel as if everything in life is a mess actually develop a messy look themselves, with angry red lesions on their face and scaling showing through their unkempt hair. Their outward appearance can certainly benefit from improved centering through achieving a state of inner calm and quiet. This doesn't mean that most people with dandruff suffer from emotional distress. It is simply a reminder that if all other treatments are not working, emotional status is another area to consider, which is a process that requires both your own introspection and some perspective from a practitioner who is skilled at helping people identify, work through, and resolve emotional issues.

My Approach

Start slowly with a conservative approach to treatment. A person who has had mild dandruff that clears completely with occasional use of over-the-counter shampoos may not need to become involved with the program I am describing here. But if the condition continually returns and worsens, it is time to progress to stronger treatment.

First, build a healthy foundation. If there is history consistent with yeast issues, I suggest a low yeast diet. If that does not help enough, I use the measures described earlier to reduce yeast in the intestinal tract and replace it with organisms normally found in the intestines. At the same time, I suggest changing the balance of essential fatty acids toward the anti-inflammatory oils.

From there, I fine tune the program, looking for foods to eliminate that could be aggravating the seborrhea or other symptoms. Food allergies are easier to develop when yeast causes inflammation in the intestines, acting as if it is poking tiny holes in the intestinal walls. This leads to what has been termed "leaky gut," a condition discussed in Chapter 11. Soon even more commonly eaten foods aggravate your immune system, and thus your digestive system and other organs in your body become targets of the process. You will have to avoid the other foods that trigger a response as well until your digestive system settles down, the barrier is restored, and you can re-educate your immune system to ignore such foods (*see Illustration page 181*).

Some people prefer to use essential oils (fragrant, potent, plant-derived oils not to be confused with essential fatty acids) such as tea tree oil, thyme oil, or rosemary oil as topical anti-yeast products. These also bring about improvement, but have the disadvantage of having a strong odor and a slight tendency to cause allergic rashes. After being diluted, they may be rubbed into the skin or incorporated into natural shampoos.

Therapeutic shampoos can be added for additional improvement. Zinc pyrithione shampoos, such as the classic Head and Shoulders, are effective in mild cases. Zinc pyrithione may have mild suppressive effects on the immune system response. These often have a blue-green color. Selenium-containing shampoos are more effective for some. A stronger, 2.5 percent selenium shampoo is dispensed by prescription only. Ketoconazole shampoo is an antifungal that is now available. Tar shampoos are an old standby for treatment of dandruff and other scaly red conditions. Their mode of action is not well known. Their disadvantage is the smell (like road tar) and the fact that they can stain clothing. Pine tar is an option as well.

What I Avoid, and When I Prescribe Specific Medications

When seborrhea is more severe, it involves the eyebrows, forehead, and creases beside the nose. Cortisone and more powerful topical steroids will quickly calm this down, but the condition will return just as quickly when the medication wears off. If the immune system has been suppressed by steroids, the seborrhea may return with a vengeance, since the yeast in the skin grows more during the time of reduced immune system control. The temptation is to use a stronger cortisone to gain control, and this ratcheting up the strength of the cortisone continues because the less powerful cortisones stop working. The problem, well known to dermatologists, is that use of stronger cortisone products for a month or more leads to permanent atrophy, or thinning of the skin on the face. When that happens, the skin loses its normal ridging pattern, and appears shiny. Also, the thinner skin exposes the capillary blood vessels just under the surface, and the skin takes on a permanent reddish appearance, with fine blood vessels showing through. This is especially pronounced when the more powerful fluorinated steroids are used. Steroid acne can also result, and I have seen a number of patients who appear to be addicted to steroid cream use on the face, since they worsen immediately upon stopping the product; they therefore find it difficult to discontinue use of the cream.

Oral Anti-yeast Medications

Nystatin is probably one of the safest anti-yeast medications. Since it works by causing the wall around new yeast cells to be defective, the result is that yeast cell contents dump into the intestinal tract as the integrity of the yeast cell wall is broken. However, in patients who are already sick from yeast, contact with all those "yeast cell innards" can cause quite an aggravated reaction. Even building the dose up slowly can result in a number of reactions; therefore, I usually start out by recommending gentler, more natural supplements to reduce the yeast population before initiating Nystatin. It has turned out that the gentler remedies often do the job, so I rarely need to progress to the Nystatin treatment. Another problem that my colleagues and I observed years ago was actually related to Nystatin's effectiveness. A number of patients on the yeast-free diet figured out that by taking the Nystatin, they could get away with cheating on the diet. Eventually, the Nystatin would stop working. I observed more than one case where there was an initial improvement of a long-persistent symptom that finally disappeared on the yeast program with Nystatin, only to reappear after discontinuing the program. The problem in this case was that re-instituting the Nystatin did not help the second time it was prescribed.

Ketoconazole has a small but definite potential for causing liver toxicity. Lasting serious damage occurs only about once in 50,000 cases. It is effective, in part because it is actually excreted in the sweat ducts that are part of the same structure on the skin as where the yeast lives. So it is an effective medication for resistant cases in which everything else has already being done. Treatment-resistant strains of yeast replace the sensitive strains when the diet still favors abundant growth of yeast in the intestines. The resistant strains grow to the extent that the diet and conditions allowed prior to treatment. The FDA has recently restricted the use of ketoconazole from to only severe fungal infections that have become resistant to other medications.

Diflucan (fluconazole) is a drug that I think of as one of the most powerful against yeast available in this country. If you use it without also making dietary changes, and as a result get resistant yeast overgrowth, there is nothing else stronger left to try. Also, there are rare but severe side effects from this drug, including liver damage. I do not understand why some physicians use this drug casually. I still see patients who were treated with Diflucan for a few weeks, without any change in diet, whose symptoms and problems come back a few days after stopping the medication. Unfortunately, repeat treatment does not achieve results as effective as the first time, possibly because a Diflucan-resistant population of yeast is growing back. I believe these are important medications that should be saved until an individual is on a low-yeast diet, and has done everything else to reduce their yeast population as much as possible. Then, it can be a powerful tool as the "final punch" to knock out the yeast dominance. It also should be reserved for future use, in case subsequent more severe life threatening yeast infections develop.

Summary

Dandruff is a problem because of its visibility, persistence, and recurrence. Most conventional therapy, such as shampoos and topical corticosteroids, only deal with the organism and the reaction that is happening locally in the skin. In this chapter, I've explained how to deal with the other half of the equation: the generation of a specific attack against the yeast in the follicle, which is the root cause of the inflammation. The attack on yeast in the follicle is related to the amount of yeast and yeast byproducts (as well as mold) in the digestive system and elsewhere in the body. Making vast changes in the body's relationship to yeast and mold can make fast changes in the presence of seborrheic dermatitis. Changes in the type of essential fatty acids consumed, such as increasing the relative amount of omega-3 essential fatty acids eaten, can also improve seborrhea. When the condition is severe, addressing these underlying causes can make it easier for medical treatment to be effective, and can reduce the amount of medication needed.

CHAPTER 14
EXPLAINING ECZEMA

Joyce's Eczema

Joyce came to see me with a rash that, for the past several months, had been becoming steadily worse, and had only improved with oil applications. She also had a history of hay fever. When I saw the rash inside of her elbows, it was easy to make the diagnosis of eczema.

She described having a balanced healthy diet, but her bottle of red wine each week alerted me to a possible problem either with yeast or with the sulfites which sometimes are present as a preservative in red wine. I placed her on a yeast-eliminating diet plus a supplement regimen to control the yeast population. I also gave her a supplement to help break down the sulfites.

When she returned, her rash had improved, but the other results she described nearly knocked me off my chair. I had not taken a complete history of her other systems, and did not know that she had had knee surgery three years previously, with subsequent pain and swelling in both of her knees. She had been getting acupuncture treatments for her knees, which gave her relief for a week or so after the treatment. After she began my program, she lost an inch of circumference from each swollen knee! Instead of slowly walking down stairs in pain, she was able to run down the stairs.

That was proof to me that the yeast was causing a whole body inflammatory allergic reaction. When the yeast was brought under control, not only did her eczema improve, but so, too, did her inflamed knees.

Overview of Atopic Dermatitis (Atopy)

Classical eczema is also known as atopic dermatitis (AD), a medical condition in which patches of skin become red, rough, and inflamed, especially in characteristic areas such as inside the elbows and behind the knees. It may be widespread and cover the entire body, and is often accompanied by a secondary infection. Eczema frequently starts in infancy and early childhood, clears, and then reoccurs later in life. Atopic dermatitis is often associated with a personal history of hay fever or asthma, and a family history of AD, hay fever, or asthma. There are other forms of eczema as well, associated with a contact allergy to particular substances, or repeated irritation, such as constant exposure to water and detergents in the case of hand eczema. The family relationship in eczema indicates that there are certain genetically transmitted characteristics that make a person more likely to develop this condition. Some of those characteristics have been discovered recently and will be discussed later in this chapter.

Unfortunately, eczema, similarly to asthma, is becoming more common among children, with some reports stating that 3-21 percent of people will have eczema at some time in their life. The following discussion of the various factors causing eczema, illustrates some of the reasons this condition is becoming more common, including accumulated defects that are passed from one generation to the next.

There is certainly evidence that environmental factors influence this condition, and the largest environmental intake, by weight, is food. Even conservative experts in the field of atopy (the genetic tendency to develop allergies) would probably agree that there is a subset of atopic diseases in which foods aggravate the condition.

Stepping back for an overview, the immune system has the daunting task of determining what is self and what is foreign, and mounting a reaction against the foreign material to remove it from the system. The history of immunology reveals layers of cellular and biochemical reactions that are constantly being uncovered as our depth of knowledge increases. From a systems approach, these reactions require a delicate balance for optimal function at any level. Likewise, they can be thrown off by "noise" in the system at any level. The nature of "progress" in our civilization since the beginning of the industrial age has been a proliferation of noise at every systemic level imaginable. For example, preservation of crops and food products comes with a heavy chemical price. Tens of thousands of new chemicals have entered our environment in our soil, food, and even food containers. The proliferation of these environmental toxins is exhausting the enzymes that break down toxic wastes, and diminishing our ability to tolerate these chemicals.

Electromagnetic signals in the air have the potential to disrupt our bodies' reactions at the electro chemical level. In addition, psychological and emotional stresses of our fast-paced world throw more noise into the system, even if only to distract us from the normal process of focusing on food and hunger to release digestive enzymes. The digestive process is severely compromised when we eat on the run, while conducting business, or while watching television—all of which have become common practice. All of these factors increase the chance that reactive foods will be the "noise" in the system that precipitates atopy.

By understanding the causes of atopic dermatitis, it is easier to decide which treatment and avoidance is necessary to gain control of the disease. Some of the outstanding symptoms of atopic dermatitis are dryness, itching, and scaling of the skin. There seems to be a tendency for the condition to spiral out of control once the dryness and itching begin. Because washing, especially washing with soap and hot water, removes the oils from the skin and causes drying, it is especially important to avoid excessive washing and drying of the skin in cases of atopic dermatitis. Many people believe they need a shower or bath every day, but for people with atopic dermatitis (especially in the winter when it is cold outside and the humidity of the indoor air is very low), bathing on a daily basis can start the process of extreme skin dryness and itching.

Itching and Scratching

One of the main features of eczema is itching, which can at times be severe. The itching often comes and goes without any obvious reason. The natural response for most people is to scratch where it itches. The scratching causes irritation and thickening of the skin and often leads to cuts or breaks, which then develop secondary infections.

This can be a real problem for patients with atopic dermatitis, because it leads to scratching that causes a breakdown of the normal skin barrier and creates opportunities for staphylococcus and streptococcus to infect the erosions and cracks that open the skin. The skin normally puts out its own powerful anti-microbial compounds, collectively known as "defensins"; recent studies have shown that people with eczema have a problem making these defensins, which makes them more susceptible to staph and strep infections of the skin. Those two organisms can act as super antigens, triggering as many as 20 percent of the lymphocytes to enter a reactive mode. This is very different from other foreign antigens, which might activate only a small fraction of a percent of the lymphocytes. So dryness and itching leads to cracking and secondary infection that leads greater inflammation and more itching and scratching. It's no wonder that this is such an annoying chronic disorder.

Most people do not wash their hands before they rub and scratch an itchy area. As a result, they are going around touching and sampling the various chemicals and bacteria in their environment and are rubbing these various chemicals and bacteria into their skin as they touch and scratch. This can lead to more sensitivities and allergies. So breaking the scratching and itching cycle is an important component of improving the skin.

I often joke with eczema patients, suggesting that I'm going to prescribe handcuffs to help stop the damage from scratching. They laugh, because the truth is, they know it would probably require an extreme measure such as handcuffing to stop them from scratching. And worse, they know that they would probably find some other way to scratch, even if their hands were handcuffed to the wall. This is important to remember, because repeated scratching sometimes becomes a nervous habit that continues even when there is no itch. This habit can even become similar to an addiction, with such deep roots that willpower alone will not stop it. It can also aggravate the entire cycle and cause the eczema to return. Although some people can break this scratching pattern by sheer determination, others need to resort to prayer or to working with a skilled therapist or support group such as one might use for stopping smoking, alcohol use, or overeating.

If you have eczema, a valid excuse might seem to be that you would stop scratching if you stopped itching. This is where another vicious cycle comes into play, because clearly itching will come and go with this condition, and scratching will make it worse. So the paradox is that you need to stop the scratching (whether or not you itch), to break this vicious cycle. Although I advocate a natural approach, for some people use of anti-itch medications, when the itch is most severe, is necessary to help them stop scratching. I know this statement may offend some readers who oppose any use of corticosteroids and antihistamines. In my experience, following weeks of treatment to clear someone's skin, it is important to provide tools to prevent a night of digging and scratching that can open the skin, thus requiring an additional several weeks to heal, therefore aggravating the entire cycle of infection, itching, and scratching.

First, you need to develop a strategy to prevent the vicious cycle of infection in areas of scratched broken skin leading to more itching. Try a frozen gel pack from the freezer, or ice cubes, and place them over the itchy area to get relief. You can also control the urge to scratch by immediately starting a deep breathing exercise, which you have practiced in times when you are not itching. Bring yourself to a state of calm and inner focus. While in temporary control of the itching and scratching, you can decide your next steps to gain long-term control of the itching and the eczema.

The steps may include the use of natural anti-itch substances such as Quercetin or Stinging Nettle. Calming the itch may require natural creams. Or in severe cases, control of the itch may require topical or oral antihistamines. Some people do well with topical anesthetics. Although I try to avoid topical steroids, they may be useful at the time of severe itching to break the itch cycle, as long as they are not used regularly for this purpose. During times that the itch is sufficiently controlled, you can focus well enough to list all the possible causes that may have triggered this episode. There may be a giant emotional conflict that is silently exploding inside you. Or you may need to take further action, such as eliminating some food or exposure, or to seeing your dermatologist or other health professional to determine the likely cause and how to reverse the outbreak.

Keeping the Skin Moist

When itching starts, there are a number of natural methods that can be used to control it, including less frequent bathing and discontinued use of soaps, which have been discussed in Chapter 9.

Applying ice cubes often breaks the itch because of the strong sensation it provides. Hydrating the skin by wearing wet clothing, followed by the application of a cream or ointment to seal in the moisture, can help. Mild anti-inflammatory creams such as those containing chamomile can also help.

Another way that you can keep your skin moist is by drinking enough water. Because eczema causes excessive water loss through the skin, extra consumption of water is required to replace that loss. This lesson was illustrated by a patient who had a problem with dry scaly skin. He was otherwise in good health and I had done everything possible to help him control his eczema through nutrition; however, he avoided drinking water because he was afraid he would have to wake up too often during the night to urinate. One day he returned with his skin clear of the dryness and scaling. He had decided that clear skin was a greater priority than a few nighttime trips to the bathroom, and had begun to drink sufficient water.

Understanding Eczema

A number of scientific discoveries in the past few years have added greatly to our understanding of this complex set of conditions that presents as eczema. The conditions include:

- Defects in the skin barrier that disrupt the normal protection from skin against entry of foreign materials and skin dryness resulting from water escape from the body;

- Decreased natural ability to combat common bacterial dangers such as staph infections, combined with immune system over-activation by the substances emitted by those same bacteria;

- Immune system defects of over-reaction;

- Allergic response to foods (a which is a triggering factor in about a third of the cases of eczema; the key here is not only the foods eaten, but the byproducts of those foods that actually enter the body's circulation and lymphatics, which then cause trouble);

- Mechanical factors such as scratching, which play a role in allowing an infection or foreign allergenic chemicals and materials to enter the skin;

- Mental and emotional factors, which can influence both scratching and itching.

Skin cells migrate to the surface, becoming thinner and flatter as they do. Some of the oils and other skin products are deposited between these flattened cells on the surface, and together they form a barrier. This barrier is not unlike the shingles and tar on a roof, providing a barrier to keep water out of a house and keep moisture in.

One of the components of the "tar between the shingles," (or the "mortar between the bricks") on the skin is a combination of waxes called ceramides, that form only in the uppermost layer of the skin, known as the "stratum corneum." Dr. Peter Elias, a dermatologist and scientist from San Francisco, did a lot of the early work in discovering the ceramides, finding that a combination of different ceramides worked best in creating the water vapor evaporation barrier in the skin. Since that time, a number of ceramide-containing creams have come onto the market to help with eczema. Sales and patient reports indicate that these creams can be helpful. How the creams approximate Dr. Elias's finding on the correct combination of ceramides necessary to produce a barrier may be an important factor in how helpful they are. Effects of other beneficial components for a particular individual and situation, such as anti-microbial compounds, can make a big difference in the effectiveness of these creams. Like other creams, if they contain ingredients to which you are allergic, such as fragrances, even the beneficial ceramides will not give you a positive effect.

Another defect relatively recently discovered in eczema patients is in a protein called "filaggrin." Filaggrin protein appears to have a number of different roles as its structure changes, while moving up toward the outermost layer of the epidermis. The best way to visualize how filaggrin functions as it changes is to think of the kids' toys known as Transformers. Some start out as spaceships, and by bending and moving some pieces around, can become fierce warriors. Let's carry this step further, and imagine that if we break the Transformers apart into several pieces, each of those pieces would have another set of functions. The three stages of transformation would mimic what we know about the filaggrin molecule. Imagine if one or more parts of the Transformer were defective. It would not work as a spaceship, would not fold properly into a warrior, and the parts would not do what they should as individual components.

That is the case with the defective filaggrin molecule leading to a series of defects that makes eczema more likely. Initially, the filagrrin is the main component of the structure of the granules that will lead to the uppermost barrier, known as "keratohyalin" granules. In this "profilaggrin" form, it also has a role in signaling other cells and preparing the skin cells to transform into a barrier. When the "pro-filaggrin" transforms into filaggrin, it plays a further role in forming filaments and preventing water loss. In the uppermost layer, it is broken down into amino acids that have several functions: they hold water in the upper dermis to keep it moist; maintain the acid pH of the skin; help maintain the barrier; and protect against staphylococcal infection. Defective filaggrin breakdown products expose the skin to more infections with staphylococcus and other bacteria. With the defective filaggrin, there is excessive water loss through the skin leading to the characteristic dryness and scaling. Also, foreign materials from the outside enter more easily, causing more allergies. More allergies leads to more itching, which leads to more scratching, which leads to further damage of the skin barrier and more open areas to become infected so that the vicious cycle of eczema gets off to a roaring start.

Stress and Eczema

Anita's Eczema

Anita came to me for eczema that had some resemblance to another condition related to gluten sensitivity. Here are her words:

"About four years ago when I was facing a great deal of stress, my body began to show signs of the stress both internally and externally. I broke out with several itchy rashes all over my body that had been previously diagnosed as eczema. As a result of the stress I began to look for ways to comfort myself and found myself eating white flour butter cookies with my tea before going to bed. Internally I was feeling gas, bloating, and constipation with an insane itch on my lower extremities. The rashes on my body had turned several shades darker than my skin and were prevalent and visible. They were so extreme that clothing touching the rashes caused severe pain. The itching was unbearable. I was under such distress that I finally sought a second round of medical treatment.

"When I went to Dr. Dattner, he observed the severely itchy grouped bumps on the outside of my extremities and considered gluten sensitivity. He also noticed that I developed new outbreaks of a rash after eating wheat products on various occasions. He tested me for gluten/antigenic food sensitivity and noticed the level of intestinal anti-gliadin IgA antibody was elevated in my stool, indicative of active dietary gluten and other common food sensitivity. I was taken off gluten and given digestive enzymes, a low yeast diet, and other support for my digestive tract. My itching is almost completely gone and the thick, dark areas of my skin began to calm down. When I avoid gluten, my belly no longer feels bloated, as it did before. I still eat gluten occasionally, but have lesser outbreaks afterward. My skin itching and thickening and my digestive system are much improved and no longer sensitive to the touch of my clothing.

"Thank you, Dr. Dattner, for helping me regain my health."

There are many people who experience aggravation of their eczema with stress. People often find that they scratch more when they are under stress, as they lose their ability to suppress this habit. Digestion does not work as well during times of stress, when one's thoughts are with the stress rather than with the food being eaten. Numerous studies have been done on the nervous system and immune system under stress and how they affect the skin. These studies demonstrate additional ways in which stress can lead to aggravation of eczema. Finding better ways to change the situation or how you react to the situation are keys to reducing the stress and how it affects your skin.

Dr. John Sarno, in *The Divided Mind*, describes a group of psychosomatic factors he calls "tension myositis syndrome," (TMS) which he has found to be a major cause of back pain. From his experience, eczema has a similar cause. In those patients for whom this is true, the contribution of foods to AD is harder to assess. "Stuffing" emotional pain by eating to excess or consuming problematic foods is one mechanism by which emotional stress and food can interact to trigger or exacerbate AD.

Environmental Aggravators

In a study from the United Kingdom, Dr. SM Langan found that a number of different exposures were associated with worsening of eczema. These were nylon, house dust, shampoo, sweating, swimming, exposure to unfamiliar pets, and wearing of wool clothing. Exposure to three of these seven factors increased the chance of an eczema flare. This supports the concept that the more aggravators present, the more likely eczema will break out. It also suggests that the more you reduce the aggravators, the better your skin will be if you have eczema. Another factor is sweat. Sweat can leach chemicals out of clothing, or capture dust, pollen, and other allergens from the air. All sorts of chemicals from the blood are concentrated and excreted in the sweat glands, so it is possible that this may be another source for stimulating an irritant or allergic reaction in the skin of people with eczema.

Food and Atopic Dermatitis

Some people with eczema clearly have outbreaks after certain foods. Others get better on the elimination diet, although they initially have no idea what their aggravating foods may be. Some doctors, nutritionists, and websites suggest that specific foods, such as wheat and milk, be eliminated to clear eczema. Following the suggestions to eliminate some of the more common foods associated with eczema may bring relief to some people. This kind of prescription is a little like betting on horses, choosing the more commonly eaten foods and seeing if eliminating them helps. The actual food triggers often vary greatly, not only among different eczema sufferers, but over time with each one. If you stop eating wheat because you were shown to be allergic, and you start eating a lot of corn, you will probably wind up allergic to the corn.

It is not just what food is eaten, but the degree to which it is broken down, and what actually enters the body that counts. The way the proteins in food are split apart into smaller components known as peptides, and sometimes, eventually, amino acids, determines what will be available to get into the bloodstream and lymphatics around the intestines. If digestion is incomplete, proteins are only partly broken down into larger peptides. These peptides, or chains of amino acids, may be large enough to be recognized by the immune system and trigger allergic reactions in the skin. This can happen only if the peptides can enter the circulation through a defective barrier in the intestinal wall (this is discussed further in the section in Chapter 11 on "leaky gut").

Food and food extracts influence the ratio of pro versus anti-inflammatory prostaglandins via fatty acid content and influence on fatty acid metabolism. Dietary probiotics, and the degree to which, along with diet, they influence gut flora and permeability, play a role as well. Emerging nutrigenomics research suggests that foods may influence other aspects of the digestive process and immunity as well as unknown factors, which may lead to AD. Foods also have the potential of modifying the digestive process, and influencing the kinds of immunogenic peptides that activate the immune system. Understanding the specific activities of different foods on various layers of the digestive and immune systems helps clinicians to interpret the experience of AD patients with foods in relationship to their disorder.

Food, Allergy, and IgE

Since eczema may be aggravated by multiple foods, and these foods vary over time, it would be very helpful to have a laboratory test one could rely on to determine which foods are problems. As discussed before in this book, the immune system in the body has as many branches as has the defense system for a country. Medical laboratory science has evolved to the point that we can perform specific tests to evaluate the function of specific branches of the immune system. One has to first understand which part of the immune system is involved in the inflammatory attack in eczema before deciding what branch of the immune system to test.

Current thinking is that eczema begins as an antibody-type response and later becomes more of a cellular immune response when it is chronic. The antibody-type responses are known as TH2. Many different types of antibodies can be involved with the TH2 responses. IgE testing is extremely helpful for immediate type sensitivity reactions in which people developed symptoms within minutes of exposure. This includes reactions to inhalants such as pollen, and mold leading to asthma or hives. Nutritionally-oriented physicians had found IgE testing to be much less reliable in regard to food sensitivity.

There are numerous tests of blood and of stool that provide information on what foods are eliciting a reaction. Many of these tests may be helpful in determining which foods to eliminate to achieve improved eczema. Unfortunately, none of these tests are absolutely accurate. They miss some foods that cause eczema and erroneously identify others that do not, in the individual being tested. They may, however, provide a good start by pointing out a number of foods likely to cause trouble. The gold standard is to eliminate suspected foods and challenge with them later. If there is improvement after elimination, and aggravation after reintroduction of a food, it is likely that the food is an aggregator to be avoided.

Cow's milk allergy is among the most common allergies reported. Using skin prick testing, 44.5 percent of patients with atopic dermatitis were positive for cow milk allergens; there also were positive reactions to tomato (29.41 percent), egg (28.57 percent), nuts (9.24 percent) and wheat (3.36 percent).

Patch testing has been shown to reliably identify and demonstrate food allergens in AD. A study from South Africa, with the premise that food association with atopy is irrefutable, broke food responses in atopics into two categories. The most common triggers of cutaneous symptoms are tomatoes, oranges, sweets, pineapple, chocolate, and soft drinks preserved with sulfur dioxide. These foods result in symptoms in 30 to 49 percent of children tested.

Leaky Gut

Escape of food allergens across the gut wall likely plays a role in food aggravation of AD. Likewise, the degree of intestinal permeability to dietary antigens is a crucial variable in food allergy. Most studies on food and eczema do not evaluate this leakage. I believe that this leakage of food-derived allergens across the intestinal barrier is one of the most important unrecognized factors in causing eczema. It modifies all of the results seen by simply looking at which foods are eaten, and explains why dermatologists have been so confused by the issue of food allergy for decades.

Just as disruption of the skin leads to increased permeability to external allergens, disruption of the normal barrier function in the gut resulting from inflammation or other factors leads to enhanced entry of food allergens. Variation in this permeability defect can vastly alter food allergen activation of AD, and may account for why, in one study, people who had AD and were allergic to milk were also found to be more sensitive to cereals.

Anti-inflammatory EFAs

Besides the immune factors, the dryness, the scratching, and the ability to defend against infection, there is another system in the skin that controls the potential for a breakout in AD. This system consists of oil-based signal molecules called "prostaglandins" (already discussed in Chapter 11). The ratio of the different types of prostaglandins you produce determines whether inflammation in your skin will be triggered by the slightest exposure to an allergen, or whether a significant reaction is required to do so. Prostaglandins have other signal properties as well, and were first discovered in the gland they were named for, the prostate gland. Since what you eat has a big influence on your balance of prostaglandins, and prostaglandins influence how good or bad your eczema is, I will discuss where they come from, where they exist in our cells, and what causes them to become more or less aggravating for AD.

As mentioned in Chapter 11, prostaglandins are made from particular types of oils, known as "essential fatty acids" (EFAs), which are present in specific types of food. Enzymes convert these essential fatty acids into prostaglandins. There are two types of prostaglandins that calm inflammation. PGE 1 is an anti-inflammatory signal made from gamma linoleic acid, an EFA found especially in evening primrose oil and borage oil. PGE 3 is another major anti-inflammatory prostaglandin found especially in omega-3 unsaturated fatty acids that come from fish oils from cold water fish and cold climate plants such as flaxseed. Both of these have been reported to have an anti-inflammatory effect that can benefit patients with eczema.

Therefore, another way to gain control of eczema is to increase the anti-inflammatory oils and fats in the diet and decrease the ones that lead to inflammation. Unfortunately, some enzymes in this inflammation-calming pathway are inhibited by partially hydrogenated oils and high insulin levels from excessive sugar consumption. So just taking the oils may not help if you are consuming partially hydrogenated oils and excessive amounts of sugar. Since these oils are unsaturated, they are susceptible to either oxidation or combining with other body chemicals. It makes sense to protect these essential fatty acids with fat-soluble antioxidants such as vitamin E.

Knowing more about where these EFAs are found in nature and our cells and how they are changed in the body helps us to understand how we can elicit from them the maximum power of reducing AD inflammation. They are part of the normal food chain in cold water and cold climates, where fish eat krill and plankton. "Unsaturated" oils remain as a liquid and do not turn solid at low temperatures. When we heat unsaturated oils in cooking, they literally "harden"; they turn solid when we put them back in the refrigerator. They have been chemically changed, and oxidized or saturated, by the process of heating them in the oxygen, and they no longer have the desirable anti-AD properties. Modern society imports saturated oils from warmer climates in the South, and hydrogenates oils for better shelf life and other cooking characteristics. As a result, people living in the colder parts of the globe now have a much lower ratio of omega-3 unsaturated fatty acids in their bodies than they did 100 years ago, and a greater tendency toward inflammatory conditions such as AD.

Summary

Atopic dermatitis, often called eczema, has different causes in different people. Over-drying of the skin by excessive washing is one. Rubbing and scratching aggravates the condition and leads to secondary infection that further aggravates the skin. Controlling infection and cultivating growth of a beneficial mix of microorganisms in the digestive system, skin, and overall body is helpful. Avoiding irritants and allergens in the environment and in whatever is applied to your skin is important. Food allergies and food sensitivity seem to aggravate some people with this condition. Aiding the digestive system, along with avoiding foods that can aggravate your skin are steps that can improve the overall eczema condition. Adding the right kind of essential fatty acids internally also benefits eczema and other conditions. Controlling emotional aggravators is essential. Different people have different defects and aggravators, and other specific defects are being discovered all the time. Both general and individual specific steps are necessary to free an individual from the ravages of AD.

CHAPTER 15
HIVES DON'T JUST HAPPEN

Have you ever seen red spots arise before your eyes? If they were broad red raised bumps on your skin, they were most likely hives, one of the most common biological reactions to many types of allergens.

Let's get the technical details of hives out of the way: The condition of hives, technically termed Urticaria, shows up as raised red itchy bumps that come and go within a day, often recurring day after day. They may be broad, covering large portions of an arm or other part of your body. Their borders move around over time and can appear on different areas during a given outbreak. Hives are caused by release of histamine (a chemical substances your immune system cells produce in response to foreign invaders in your body such as drugs and bacteria) and other inflammatory mediator molecules that cause the capillaries to open up and leak fluid into the tissues. Release of histamine and related molecules comes from tiny sacs known as vesicles located in mast cells (immune system cells in the tissues that are filled with granules containing histamine and other mediators) and basophils (a type of white blood cell). The release of histamine produces the typical swelling that is seen in the skin in hives. Other symptoms, including joint pain, abdominal pain, and disturbance of other organs, may accompany hives.

Why Do We Get Hives?

Think of hives as a kind of warning red flasher on your skin, similar to the warning light on the dashboard of your car. It is telling you that something is occurring, usually on the *inside*, but it does not tell you what. If you coordinate the onset of the hives together with exposures to foods, medications, conditions, and/or infections that preceded it, you will begin to identify a list of possible causes. This is an important starting point for discovering and eliminating the cause of your hives. There are many different classes of causes of hives, and many diets proposed to eliminate them. The Internet is filled with such diet plans along with testimonials to their effectiveness. Without challenging the observations reported, this chapter will explore the multiple reasons specific foods may aggravate hives, beyond the reasons that are claimed. The importance of this flexibility and expansion of perspective is that it may suggest additional or different groups of foods to be eliminated by someone with hives, beyond those typically classified as urticaria aggravators. Those groupings may turn out to be more relevant to your recovery.

Hives can be caused by numerous different immunological and chemical mechanisms, including Immunoglobulin E (IgE) and IgG antibodies that cause immediate reactions. Non-immunologic causes can include drugs such as opiates and contrast media used for specialized x-ray exams. The opioids, such as codeine, appear to cause hives by directly causing the granules in mast cells to release histamine into the tissues. Hives can also develop as a result of cold or heat exposure or from pressure to the skin.

Medical literature suggests that a cause is found for urticaria in anywhere from a few percent to up to 50 percent of cases. In many cases there is more than one cause. A longtime lecture at the American Academy of Dermatology, was "Urticaria: Seek at least two causes." Some physicians give up entirely on ever finding the cause, so they give long courses of antihistamines to calm down the reaction. Dermatologists, allergists, and other physicians prove their mettle by the detective work they do to find out what factors bring about the condition in a given individual.

Food Allergens and Hives

There are many foods (especially shellfish, tree nuts, milk, and fruit) that can cause hives.

Some foods contain high amounts of histamine, and some of these cause histamine release as well. The lists of which foods have the highest histamine levels differ greatly depending on who is making the list; however, some of the same foods seem to show up consistently. High-histamine foods include Baker's yeast, strong moldy cheeses, spinach, trout, sardines, tuna, tomato, avocado, coconut, and fermented foods such as sauerkraut, soy, and red wine. Interestingly, Baker's yeast and moldy cheeses both strongly aggravate intestinal Candida overgrowth issues (which aggravate leaky gut) and allergic reactions because they open the gate for food allergens to escape into the blood supply. So there may be aggravation of hives by these foods, as well other foods listed as high histamine (such as mushrooms, vinegar, and yeasty cakes and breads), which suggests the need to follow a yeast-free diet rather than just a low-histamine diet.

It is important to understand that observations and interpretations about why certain foods could lead to urticaria should be expanded so that you can see how they overlap with other interpretations. For example, histamine-containing foods are suspected to contribute to the excess histamine that is released in the body. Milk products, and especially cheese (which is high in histamine), are common allergens, and could cause hives on a dairy allergy (casein, whey) basis. Hormones or antibiotics in the milk could be the aggravator. The mold in blue cheese (a high-histamine food) is very strong, and could aggravate on the basis of being part of the fungus family, related to yeasts in the digestive system.

Other foods, such as chocolate, alcohol, fish, shellfish, and strawberries, are reported to release histamine. It should be noted that shellfish may also contain a variety of human microbes and pathogens, since they are filterers in estuaries where sewage may run off. So shellfish can also initiate allergic reactions because of the live or dead microbes in their guts. Red wine also can aggravate by being a source of sulfites, or because of its high yeast byproduct content. Alcohol breakdown products such as acetaldehyde interfere with the breakdown of histamine by the "diamine oxidase" (DAO) enzyme, thus keeping histamine levels high. Histamine is normally broken down by two different enzymes, diamine oxidase (DAO), and histamine-N-methyltransferase (HNMT). Conditions and foods that diminish the effectiveness of DAO can cause histamine levels to be higher, and thus lead to hive formation. Several medications including chloroquine, cycloserine, and clavulanic acid inhibit this enzyme, as do detergents added to medications to make oils soluble.

Hives from food allergy may be caused by anything that initiates the cycle of absorption of undigested foodstuff. A common trigger for this cycle is yeast overgrowth in the digestive tract. Yeast is not the only cause of hives, but it is a common condition that leads to allergies to foods that are eaten (the sequence of yeast overgrowth leading to leaky gut leading to excess escape of food allergens into the blood is discussed at length in other chapters). Baker's yeast is listed as having one of the highest levels of histamine, and along with other high yeast foods, is often listed as a cause of hives.

We are a high sugar-eating culture, consuming 140 pounds of sugar per person per year. That is over a third of a pound of sugar per person per day. Combine that with an antibiotic to kill normal bacteria, and the yeast population in the intestines can have a reproduction party and take over. When they do, they irritate the intestinal wall; with this irritation, some folks will begin absorbing foods they should have kept out. Soon the immune system is reacting against more and more things you eat every day and you are breaking out in hives. Reversing this whole process in the digestive system can calm down chronic hives, as in the case below.

Cleo's Hives

Cleo had bothersome recurrent hives every day, despite being treated by her allergist with two different antihistamine drugs. She was really frustrated about taking so much medicine, and yet still having hives. She was frustrated enough so to seek out my care. I discovered a history of exposures likely to cause a yeast overgrowth, and put her on a yeast-free diet and program designed to remove the yeast and replace it with normal bacteria. She was placed on Quercetin, a natural antihistamine; a regimen designed to eliminate environmental allergens such as essential oils; and a program to support her digestive and liver function. She began to improve, and was able to drop one of the medications, but still continued to have daily hives. As she progressed with the program, she was able to clear her hives completely, and then to stop both medicines and stay clear. In about three months, she was able to stop the supplements I had given to her and after six months, most of the restrictions were lifted, and she still remained clear of hives.

Hives may occur for more than one reason. This is emphasized to make sure that you not see only the relationships between an offending food and your outbreak; it is important to also see that the outbreak may result from relationships other than the one offered. Each interpretation will place suspicion on a group of foods related to the original food a different way. Unless you keep this perspective in mind, you may give up foods without giving up the ones that are causing your hives.

More Possible Causes

Hives can also be caused by infections, whether hidden or obvious. While researching your hives, your doctor may discover the cause to be something as surprising as parasites in the intestines. Viruses, such as those that cause colds, can also cause hives. Hepatitis B and C are sometimes discovered with a first symptom of hives. Bacterial infections, whether hidden or obvious, can also be a cause for hives. For example, infections in the teeth and jaw can cause hives. Discovering such infections in the quest of correcting hives can provide real benefit when treatment brings them under control. Suppressing such reactions with high doses of antihistamines and corticosteroids could allow these infections to hide longer and to spread further, so it is appropriate to get skilled help in discovering the underlying causes of chronic urticaria.

Similarly, any kind of a reaction to chemicals in the environment or inside the body may be an important warning sign telling you to eliminate these exposures. For that reason, I think it is important to seek out the wisdom of the body and of a skilled physician in treating this or other allergic skin reactions.

Autoimmune conditions such as arthritis and lupus are also associated with hives because of their excess immune system reactivity leading to inappropriate inflammatory attack against one's own tissues. Evaluation of such underlying conditions by a competent physician or specialist is important, especially when hives are part of a more complicated illness. You may still want to try alternative treatment to reverse underlying causes, but with a medical analysis you will have a better idea of the potential consequences of your condition, the laboratory results to measure its progress, and the medical options to use if your condition progresses to a danger point.

Some forms of urticaria are associated with the condition of deeper swelling under the skin, known as angioedema, which can cause swelling of the tongue and the back of the throat. If the swelling becomes so great that it becomes difficult to breathe, this becomes a situation for the Emergency Room. Angioedema can potentially be fatal if it obstructs your airway and prevents you from breathing. People with this condition need a thorough evaluation, and need to carry a device with

ALAN M DATTNER, MD

which to inject themselves (such as an EpiPen®) to open up a blocked airway. Some forms of angioedema can also be a sign of an underlying tumor secreting substances that open up the blood vessels. This is most likely benign, but may require removal. Diagnosis requires careful evaluation and testing.

Medications such as intravenous injected contrast dyes and opiates have been reported to release histamine. Other medications, including antibiotics such as penicillin and sulfonamides, are associated with causing hives, but this could be a results of altered intestinal flora, favoring yeast overgrowth, and allergy to the products themselves. Similarly, pain medications such as aspirin and Non-steroidal anti-inflammatory drugs (NSAIDS) may cause hives because of their interference not only with molecules of communication, but also because they irritate the intestinal barrier and inhibit secretion of the protective mucus layer that covers the barrier. Other information molecules besides histamine can also cause water to escape tiny blood vessels and cause hives, or can trigger inflammation leading to hives.

Treatment

It should be obvious from the discussion here that the recommended treatment for hives is to figure out the cause(s) and then remedy or remove them. This may involve elimination of the food or substance causing the hives, more complex treatment of chronic infection and inflammation, and/or enhancing various ways the body breaks down histamine and other mediators of hives. Acute treatment of severe hives associated with swelling of the throat usually requires injected antihistamines as well as epinephrine and other methods to reduce swelling and restore the airway. More commonly, hives are a problem because they keep coming back again and again.

Holistic treatment involves detective work with an emphasis on: food allergy; digestion and leaky gut; a healthy respect for food additives; checking for yeast sensitivity; and an intensive search for hidden drugs responsible for the reaction. It also involves choosing diets, herbs, and supplements to improve the function of organs and enzymes involved in the removal of infections, inflammation, and toxic substances contributing to the hives. Sometimes it involves addressing emotional issues and stresses related to hives outbreaks.

So part of the problem is finding the offending food, chemical, or drug. It can be more difficult if the drug was present in meat or milk that the patient ingested (as penicillin often is). Aspirin can cause problems and is chemically similar to tartrazine (a chemical used to color food, drugs, and cosmetics) and yellow dye #5, which is present in prepared foods, medications, and creams. One thing about immune system reactions is that the body magnifies its recognition biologically, so a tiny bit is all it takes to trigger a reaction. Patients sometimes tell me that they only use a little milk in their cereal and since the milk only has a minuscule amount of hormone or penicillin in it, how could it cause such a reaction? I remind them that poison ivy-sensitive individuals don't have to rub the leaf daily to have a rash; some just have to sit in the seat that the dog sat in after brushing poison ivy leaves in the woods. It doesn't take much. I was puzzled to hear that an environmentally sensitive patient of mine had reacted to the tiny bit of lidocaine I had injected as anesthesia before removing a small skin lesion, since it is rare to find anyone allergic to that anesthetic. As it turns out, most lidocaine is preserved with a very small amount of sulfites, and from her history, I knew that it must have been the miniscule amount of sulfites that were the cause of her reaction.

Some people are helped by natural antihistamines, including Quercetin (found in onion skin, apples, and various other plants). Another important natural remedy for hives is stinging nettle, *Urtica dioica*. Oddly enough, the stinging nettle plant has tiny barbs on the leaves and stems that inject histamine if you touch them against your skin, causing hive formation. Cooking or preparation of an extract from these plants produces the exact opposite reaction: the calming of hives with an anti-histamine effect.

A variety of antihistamines are available as over-the-counter and prescribed drugs. These should be considered and be available for urticaria outbreaks that cannot be controlled by elimination of foods and the use of natural products. One of the reasons to consider pharmacologic antihistamines for severe reactions is that high histamine levels block the DAO, the very enzyme that is responsible for breaking down the released histamine in the body. Severe reactions may need immediate emergency care and all the modern therapeutic methods to restore the ability to breathe. Those who know they have such reactions to certain foods or exposures should carry proper antihistamines and an EpiPen®, and should not toy with eating provocative foods. One such person I am aware of knew he was allergic to shellfish, but had a habit of eating it anyway, thinking he could throw it up later and avoid danger. He did not, and subsequently died from the reaction, despite efforts to save him. His irresponsible behavior not only killed him; it tied up the lives of those who tried to save him with ongoing lawsuits. Do not challenge yourself with foods or drugs that could cause a reaction that stops your ability to breathe. I've had patients who have dangerous allergies tell me, "I really want to try eating this food again; it's been a while since I had a reaction." This may be an outlandish suggestion, but I tell my patients, if you want to do this, do it parked outside the emergency room. If it is even remotely possible you will have a life-threatening reaction, the consequences may be more than you are willing to pay.

Summary

This chapter is not meant to be the definitive guide to self-treatment of hives. It is meant, however, to give you an important perspective that you may not obtain elsewhere, about what other exposures or foods may be related to a suspected aggravator. It also is meant to show you how the overall principle of food allergies resulting from leaky gut, discussed elsewhere in this book, often needs to be treated to calm down chronic hives. This is more than a simple food or group of foods or substances causing hives. It is about foods and medications and environmental exposures creating a condition that makes it more likely that an allergic reaction will occur. Unfortunately, this perspective is relevant but has not been adopted into general thinking among most dermatologists and allergists. Therefore, it is necessary for you to bring this perspective with you and share it with your physicians as they search for simple as well as more esoteric and dangerous causes of your condition.

CHAPTER 16
THE HEARTBREAK OF PSORIASIS

Helen's Missing Diagnosis

Helen came to me for help with her psoriasis in 1985, shortly after I began to learn about the relationship between yeast in the digestive system and the onset of psoriasis. A number of physicians in my holistic medical group had read and studied the work of Dr. C. Orion Truss, who had written a pioneering book called *The Missing Diagnosis*, about the effects of the yeast Candida albicans and its intestinal overgrowth on a wide variety of medical conditions, including psoriasis. Dr. Sid Baker was a real leader in our group on this issue, describing success in treating psoriasis patients using a diet and treatment plan that reduced yeast in the body. I had placed several patients on a yeast-free diet and anti-yeast supplements, but most of them had no improvement in their psoriasis after one month of treatment. I suggested that they abandon the treatment, and was about to stop prescribing the anti-yeast program for psoriasis for my patients, when Helen came back to see me.

Helen had rather severe and prominent psoriasis, which had improved by taking methotrexate previously prescribed by another dermatologist. She knew that methotrexate was a risky and potentially fatal drug. It works by poisoning the dividing immune system cells (lymphocytes) that cause the inflammatory reaction that leads to psoriasis. These lymphocytes are the cells that are involved in triggering the immune system to start the inflammation that leads to psoriasis. Methotrexate poisons and stops the rapidly dividing skin cells that lead to the overgrowth of the thick skin we see in psoriasis. While it stops most dividing cells, methotrexate can potentially poison the bone marrow and shut down production of the white blood cells (especially lymphocytes) needed by the immune system for fighting infection and cancers in the body. Knowing that, Helen was very motivated to stick with the yeast-free diet and program for at least six months. She returned to see me with improvements in her skin condition that equaled those that she that had gotten on methotrexate! That was quite an eye-opener for the both of us.

From then on, I explained to patients that successful treatment required a long time commitment, and does not necessarily occur in a month, or at all, in every case. But it works for some. Psoriasis is a challenge for both physician and patient, and I have seen many prominent holistic physicians who have been humbled by this condition. Perhaps that is why we now have new pharmaceutical preparations known as "biologics," which can cost over $50,000 per year, achieve success in some fraction of the patients, and have possible side effects such as life-threatening infections, skin cancer and lymphoma. This is an index of how desperate we are to control this condition, and how much therapeutic power it takes to do so.

Dan's Gums

Dan had such bad psoriasis that he was on one of the new powerful drugs derived from Vitamin A when he came to see me. Not only did he not want to be on the drug, but the drug didn't seem to be making any improvement in his skin, even after nearly four months. I suggested that he follow a yeast-free diet, and gave him supplements to reduce yeast, restore normal flora to the gut, and generally improve digestion. I also gave him supplements to reduce inflammation of the skin, including EPA-rich fish oils. I gave him nearly a dozen different supplements, all told, to see if we could make a difference in his condition. When he returned about a month later to get more supplements, he told me he had no trouble following the diet strictly. No cheating or slips on special occasions. His hands still had fine bubbles and tiny pustules all over the palms, but the rash on his body had basically cleared! I was able to find only three tiny red plaques, two of which were less than a quarter inch in diameter.

I added some supplements. He had stopped the vitamin A-like drug on his own two weeks previously, with no worsening of the improvements so far. We could assume that the drug was still in his system and still working when I saw him. It was impossible to say for sure whether the drug was a major contributor responsible for the improvement, and had taken four months to work, whether my program was just what was needed at that time to tilt him toward clearing his psoriasis, or whether my program alone fixed him. More likely, it was a combination of the drug working and the yeast-free program and supplements making it much easier for the drug to work.

Dan's teeth and gums had been in bad repair for a long time. I suspected that chronic infections in the gums, teeth, and supporting jaw were responsible for both his bad breath and for causing the pustular rash on his hands.

Psoriasis is a very visible condition that can be a real challenge to control by patients and their physicians. It usually appears as bright red thick scaly patches over pressure areas such as the elbows and knees, with scattered red lesions over the rest of the body and scalp, usually sparing the face. Sunlight may help some cases, but even the most powerful drugs may not clear others. With persistence, there is hope for control of this condition. Although most pharmacologic agents inhibit the later stages of the inflammatory process that leads to the rapid overgrowth of the upper layer of the skin, holistic therapy aims at reversing the factors of the underlying cause of this disorder. Getting at underlying causes can give longer and safer control of psoriasis.

In an era in which greater understanding of the mechanism of psoriasis has led to the development of immune system-targeted drugs to control the condition (which may cost more than a year's doctor visits for each treatment), anyone who is facing the choice of such treatment (the so-called Biologics) owes it to him or herself to read this chapter to become aware of the existence of the alternatives, to understand what other steps could enhance the benefit of this or any treatment, and possibly to reduce the dose and frequency of such potentially dangerous drugs in controlling their condition.

Understanding Psoriasis and Expanding Your Understanding of Skin Disorders

We understand a lot about psoriasis, but unfortunately not well enough to have simple, safe answers for treating it. People who want an easy answer find this very frustrating. What people do not realize is that the parts we do understand may already hold the key to treatment, if we only follow the known information to its logical conclusions.

We now know that there are many genetic variants that are responsible for both similar and different defects in biochemical reactions, even leading to the same disease. A disease develops as a consequence of a concert of factors. This stage is set by a genetic tendency to form the rapid skin thickening reaction characteristic of the disease. In psoriasis, this means a tendency for inflammation to trigger a process that causes the skin cells to divide so rapidly that they proceed from the bottom layer to the top layer of the skin in four to seven days rather than in twenty-eight days. The rapid growth of skin cells, along with the enlarged blood vessels that stimulate and support that growth, leads to the familiar thick red plaques we see in psoriasis. People without this tendency don't get psoriasis.

The other critical part of the concert is the stimulus of the inflammatory process in the skin that triggers an overgrowth reaction. There may be a series of other issues, such as leakage of material from the digestive system into the blood that is part of the stimulus that leads to psoriasis. And there may be more than one group of genetic defects combined with reactions to microorganisms and other environmental agents leading to a person's specific problem. As discussed throughout this book, the concept of a cross-reactive attack, stimulated by some food or organism in our internal environment and directed against a target in the skin, is how I understand the specific immune system attack in psoriasis or other skin inflammatory disorders. Using this thinking, bacteria doesn't have to infect the skin to cause psoriasis, but could infect somewhere else in the body, such as the throat, and stimulate psoriasis. Expanding this principle, psoriasis could be caused by other bacteria, yeast, fungi, or food in different individuals.

The concept of a disease has helped us greatly in classifying skin and medical conditions, but it breaks down when we assume that everyone progressed to that disease by a similar set of causes. We now know a disease develops from a series of genetic and environmental exposures, so that not everybody will contract the same disease in the same way. Why medicine clings so tightly to the disease theory in the face of this information, as if knowing the disease will tell you the treatment to get rid of it, is baffling to me in the context of this information on individual genetic specificity.

The Underlying Condition

Psoriasis sufferers have many similarities in the presentation of their illness at many levels. It is those similarities that make the disease model work in many cases. There are drugs and treatments that have been shown to help people in general with a given disease, like psoriasis, and this has been the case over many years. Many of the effective treatments, however, are aimed at the last steps of the inflammation process. "So what is wrong with that, if the condition seems to go away?" you ask. The problem remains that the underlying condition is not changed, so the symptoms can reoccur at any moment.

Let me give you an example. Were you ever very angry at someone, displaying an angry face, and someone else told you to just put on a smile? Sometimes that smile worked, and you felt better. But more often than not, the angry feelings resurfaced when the person with whom you were angry said or did something related to what provoked your feelings in the first place. The only thing you changed was the face you put on, and not what was happening inside you. Let's say that instead, you were given a powerful tranquilizer to calm you down, so that your emotions were so dulled that not much bothered you, including your anger. That is what we do to the immune system when we give a big dose of steroids. The problem there is that if a big stressor such as a serious infection comes along that needs your body's swift response, you won't be able to meet the challenge with your adrenals, which have been shut down by the steroids. The same thing is true for your immune system. Knocking out your immune system with steroids or the new biologic agents so that you don't have the inflammatory response needed to produce psoriasis may also knock out the immune response necessary to defend against TB, lymphoma, or viruses that eat your brain. A rare condition developing in a few patients with psoriasis being treated with biologics is called progressive multifocal leukoencephalopathy (PML), and is caused by the "JC virus" that many people carry; the virus is innocuous under normal conditions, but can cause disease when the immune system is suppressed. Unfortunately, recurrence of latent tuberculosis and development of lymphoma problems have also occasionally been observed when the new biologic agents are directed against the immune system for psoriasis.

If you are trolling the Internet for information about psoriasis, one person may say it's caused by an immune system T-cell attack, another one may say it's caused by the release of certain information molecules, and still another site may say something else altogether. It's difficult to get a good perspective of all of the possible causes involved at different points in the development of psoriasis. Many of these causal factors may be operating at the same time. Here are just a few of the hypothesized causes:

1. An immune system T-cell attack against something in the upper layers of the skin. Except for strep, as discussed below, what causes this attack is almost never identified, and is rarely investigated in modern medicine. It is felt to be too hard to identify. Identification is indeed very difficult because the cause varies in different individuals.

2. Release and activation of certain cytokines, prostaglandins, and other molecular factors of inflammation. TNF alpha is one of those mediators involved in this immune system attack that has been targeted by modern drugs.

3. Elevation of anti-microbial peptides in the skin.

4. Rapid acceleration of division of the cells at the bottom of the epidermis, causing rapid growth of the upper skin layer, making it thicker, with a great increase in shedding of scales.

5. Enlargement of the blood vessels in the upper dermis, supplying the blood and nutrients for this rapid growth, and causing the visible redness, and loss of heat, when it is widespread.

6. In some cases, microorganisms in the gut either aggravate inflammation by releasing endotoxins, or by promoting an autoimmune climate. Dr. Dan Littman at NYU Medical Center showed that a particular species of intestinal bacteria called segmented filamentous bacteria could cause lymphocytes to become TH 17 lymphocytes, the subset of immune system cells associated with autoimmune responses such as psoriasis.

One well-known trigger for certain forms of psoriasis is the bacteria beta hemolytic streptococcus. As a result of these strep infections, some people produce oval lesions called "guttate psoriasis," which covers their chest. This can be improved by treatment with appropriate antibiotics such as penicillin. Some people with psoriasis have positive cultures for strep or their blood has antibodies against strep, indicating that they have had or still have a recent infection. I believe that it is worth being screened for such infections if you have any suspicion of infection. It seems that people with certain transplantation antigen types are much more susceptible to strep-induced psoriasis than others.

As discussed earlier in the case report, Candida overgrowth syndrome can lead to psoriasis as well. That leads to leaky gut, and allergen exposure to certain intestinal bacteria in the digestive system that get into the blood and lymphatics.

The two organisms mentioned above, Streptococcus and Candida, aggravate psoriasis by different mechanisms. I believe that there are a host of other organisms, including different species of bacteria, yeast, fungi, and viruses, which live on or inside us. We call this group of microorganisms our microbiome. Our microbiome usually lives in harmony with us, but it has the capability to infect us. Worse, it has the capability to trigger the unfortunate immune system attack directed against our own skin tissues that initiates psoriasis in susceptible individuals. Searching for and eliminating these specific inciting organisms and their allergenic traces is potentially very important in inhibiting the psoriasis reaction. Similarly, there may also be chemicals that incite this reaction that need to be removed from the body and the diet and environment. It is also likely that certain pathologic bacteria in our colons can incite psoriasis via their endotoxins. They may not be a problem unless they migrate backward into the small intestine and their endotoxins are absorbed across a leaky gut. Furthermore, organisms living in the skin or hair follicles may create a target for cross-reactive attack (e.g., yeast living in the hair follicles).

There seems to be an aggravation of psoriasis among alcoholics, who both damage their liver with drinking alcohol and take in large amounts of yeast byproducts. It makes sense to reduce or eliminate drinking and to support the liver with herbs and herbal extracts such as milk thistle. This is not simple to do, because alcoholics sometimes drink even more to deal emotionally with having "the heartbreak of psoriasis."

Therapies to Help Control Psoriasis

Topical vitamin D products are effective in psoriasis. Vitamin D not only supports the immune system, but more relevant to psoriasis, adequate levels of vitamin D is necessary to prevent autoimmune disorders. Both calcipotriene and calcitriol (synthetic derivatives of vitamin D) are available by prescription for a price. They are also thought to work in psoriasis by reducing the proliferation of skin cells, or keratinocytes.

Therapy using sunlight or artificial light sources has long been a mainstay in the treatment of psoriasis. Although ultraviolet light has immunosuppressive capabilities which may calm down psoriasis, it is interesting to speculate that the local production of vitamin D in the skin and its multiple actions in calming psoriasis also play an important role in the ability of light to calm down psoriasis lesions. The classic light therapy included application of tar products beforehand, often overnight, and then treatment of the skin with ultraviolet light. Tar makes the skin more sensitive to the sun and enhances the effects of ultraviolet light.

In the 1970s, pre-treatment of the skin with plant-derived photosensitizers known as "Psoralens" was combined with exposure to long-wave ultraviolet light (UVA) and the treatment became known as PUVA. Although it was effective, it did cause an increased number of skin cancers. This should not be done on your own because exposure beyond the proper energy range can cause sunburn and aggravation of the psoriasis, as well as production of more skin cancers. Also, damage to the eyes can occur unless eye protection precautions are taken, not only during treatment, but afterward while the psoralens are still in your system. Even in a clinic that calibrates light sources and carefully measures the increase in light energy that you can safely tolerate, something as simple as changing a light bulb (to a new and therefore stronger light that is not worn out) can cause an unexpected burn.

A number of creams and topical applications can be helpful in psoriasis. Just applying a strong emollient ointment such as Vaseline or an olive oil, coconut oil, or Shea butter preparation over wet skin can have some calming effect. If that application is made with an anti-inflammatory essential oil such as ginger or rosemary, it may have a greater affect. Cayenne pepper extracts have been used to dampen the itching in psoriasis. Of course, potent topical steroids can be used to reduce both the itching and the lesions, but their effect does not last long and the skin requires even stronger steroids to get the same effect subsequently.

Creams containing chemicals known as fumarates can also be helpful. Fumarates are chemicals that come from the plant Fumitory. They are derived from an "organic" acid that is part of the major metabolic pathway of the body, the TCA cycle. Fumarates can also be taken internally, but they have a number of problematic side effects including inducing flashing diarrhea, and damage to the liver and kidneys. Unfortunately, there have been a few recent reports of patients with multiple sclerosis developing PML (progressive multifocal leukoencephalopathy, mentioned in the previous section) after taking fumarates internally for long periods of time. It is important to monitor function of the liver and kidneys as well as blood count during use of fumaric acid or fumarates.

Psoriasis has many similarities to seborrheic dermatitis. Indeed, there are some forms of severe seborrheic dermatitis with thick scaling in the scalp that are hard to distinguish from psoriasis and are termed sebopsoriasis. For that reason, all the suggestions for lowering yeast in the diet and in the gut, repairing leaky gut, avoiding food allergens, getting the bowels moving regularly, and supporting the liver are all important in the care of psoriasis. Rebalancing essential fatty acids with a predominance of omega-3 unsaturated fatty acids such as fish oil and flaxseed oil has also been shown to be effective in improving psoriasis. These changes have been discussed elsewhere.

Another dietary manipulation that improves psoriasis in some people involves eating a diet that moves the pH of the body in an alkaline direction, as measured by urine and saliva pH. Testing can be done by touching pH paper to the tongue or to the urine. Reaching a pH of 7.0 and above at least part of the time indicates you are going in the right direction. The change can be made by eating abundant green vegetables, especially leafy vegetables that are juiced, steamed, or raw. Such a diet is also beneficial because it avoids major allergens such as wheat and dairy. Avoidance of meat, especially that of mammals (which are similar to our own tissues), seems to be another important way to avoid the autoimmune response of psoriasis. Pork products are especially suspicious in this regard, as the meat is most similar to our own and thus more likely to provoke an attack against our own skin. Of course, following a diet that avoids one's own food sensitivities, with rotation of food, is most important.

Summary

There are many different treatments that can be combined to gain some control over psoriasis. These include topical therapeutic emollients, careful sunlight exposure, an anti-inflammatory alkaline-rising diet, support of the digestive process and liver function, omega-3 essential fatty acids, and anti-inflammatory herbs. Identification and treatment of aggravating microorganisms in the body such as Candida and Streptococcus can bring great improvement. Reduction of stress is crucial for some people. For many people, such as Cindy, whom we met at the beginning of the chapter, six months may be required for the dietary and other more gentle techniques to take effect. Strict adherence maybe required in some people.

If these steps do not accomplish sufficient control, added medication and other treatments may be required in lesser amounts because of the partial control that they can attain. Vitamin D ointment and steroid creams can be helpful for short-term relief. Light treatments combined with tar or psoralens can bring further relief. Potent chemotherapy medications such as methotrexate and the Biologics have potential serious and fatal side effects, but they may seem like a sensible choice if accompanying psoriatic arthritis begins developing despite other efforts, and threatens to cripple you from being able to perform normal activities for the rest of your life. It may also make sense if you cannot live with the appearance of widespread psoriasis. These drugs are often expensive and require active monitoring by someone who is familiar with their use. Their power, cost, and danger are a measure of the power and challenge of this sometimes elusive skin condition known as psoriasis. Remember that psoriasis has many contributing causes at different levels, and can be a challenge to the most seasoned conventional and alternative practitioners, so do not give up easily. It takes years to develop the condition, so don't expect it to go away in a few weeks.

CHAPTER 17

ENVIRONMENT, THE SKIN, AND THE BIG PICTURE

There is a vital relationship between the health of the skin on our bodies and the "skin" of the planet Earth. Both skins are very thin surfaces compared to the diameter of the entire body. The distance from the bottom of the deepest ocean to the highest flights into the stratosphere is about one five-hundredth the diameter of the earth. The depth of the dermis and epidermis of the skin is roughly one-hundredth the diameter of the body at the level of the chest. Both receive heat and minerals from within and from the outside. Both have all the dynamics of an interface (When there's an interface, there is a transition between two different areas, including transport between one boundary and another. It might be deer living at the edge of a field in the woods or bacteria living on top of your skin or transfer of water between the earth and atmosphere or between your skin and the atmosphere.). When people study interfaces, they find similarities between our skin and the earth's boundaries (*see Illustration page 227*).

Much of this book has detailed the relationship of the health of one's body to the health of the skin. This chapter expands that relationship to show how the health of your skin is in fact dependent on the health of what is all around you, environmentally and beyond.

When we dump toxic material onto the Earth's skin, it gets into our food, water, air, possessions, and body, so we're also dumping toxic material on our own skin. The health of this narrow layer of soil, plants, beings, and air affects all life on Earth, and subsequently the health of all humans.

We have a great opportunity before us: to champion the health of the "skin" of the planet on which we live. My larger goal in including this chapter is to plant a seed of change to improve health and well-being by improving conditions on the surface of the earth, which will then help to heal our own skin. Keeping our skin healthy would be much easier if it were easier to avoid being exposed daily to toxic materials that aggravate it.

Illustration
Parallel between Skin and the Earth's Skin

Are there similarities between my body and the earth? Our skin and the outer layer of the Earth have similarities, in that they both have the characteristics of surfaces. Whatever contaminates the surface of the Earth is bound to contaminate man and his body. This illustration points out some of the many parallels. We cannot have healthy skin unless we have a clean environment, or at least know enough about the contamination to be able to identify, avoid, and remedy the damage.

Parallel between Skin & Earth's Skin (surface)

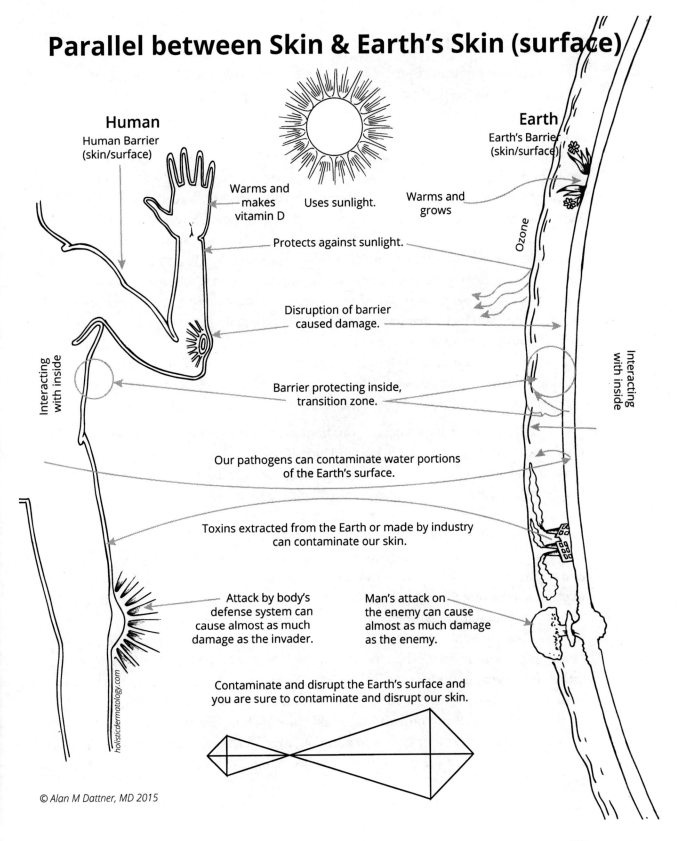

Human
Human Barrier
(skin/surface)

Warms and makes vitamin D

Uses sunlight.

Warms and grows

Earth
Earth's Barrier
(skin/surface)

Ozone

Protects against sunlight.

Disruption of barrier caused damage.

Interacting with inside

Interacting with inside

Barrier protecting inside, transition zone.

Our pathogens can contaminate water portions of the Earth's surface.

Toxins extracted from the Earth or made by industry can contaminate our skin.

Attack by body's defense system can cause almost as much damage as the invader.

Man's attack on the enemy can cause almost as much damage as the enemy.

holisticdermatology.com

Contaminate and disrupt the Earth's surface and you are sure to contaminate and disrupt our skin.

© Alan M Dattner, MD 2015

227

The Big Picture Problem

We have just come from an era with a Cowboy "wide open space" mentality, where people saw the world as so big it would absorb, neutralize, and scatter anything we dumped, burned, produced, or sold. Perhaps that was true before the Industrial Age. But we are now finding that our planet is more like a ship: what we burn in the engine room, we breathe on the poop deck. Dirty coal burned in China pollutes the air in California. Radioactive Iodine being released from the Fukushima reactor in Japan gets into our thyroids via our fish and the seaweed around our sushi. Neurotoxic and carcinogenic pesticides banned in the U.S. are sold to farmers in Central America, wind up on our shelves in the produce we eat, and ultimately accumulate in our fat, organs, and skin. Fluorocarbon propellants in our spray cans widen the hole in the ozone layer of the atmosphere that filters out harmful UV rays, meaning a greater chance of getting sunburn while standing on the surface of the Earth. The incidence of skin cancer, and especially the potentially lethal melanoma, appears to increase significantly every decade. The sun feels hotter than when we were young. No longer can we separate the condition of the skin of our bodies from the condition of the skin of our planet. We need some sanity regarding what is dumped into our environment.

The multitude of chemicals in our homes, workplaces, water supply, atmosphere, and food contribute to allergic, inflammatory, and autoimmune conditions of the skin. It may take years for the damage to accumulate, so it is hard to identify the chemical culprits. Observing changes after different exposures may give valuable hints, such as headaches after new carpets, or itching after a new cosmetic. Unfortunately, the damage from environmental toxins accumulates slowly and it may take years to cause illness and require decades of studies to prove the cause and effect relationship (look at cigarettes, for example). Elevated levels of toxins and questionable substances added to our foods and other products as a result of industry-influenced government regulating agencies are likely to have harmful health effects on some people at a later date. Worse, some companies become aware of the damage their products can cause and hide that information for years rather than trying to understand how to identify and protect those who might be harmed. In Chapter 9, we looked at a number of chemical preservatives with weak hormonal effects that not only can cause skin allergy, but may also contribute to internal cancer in the unlucky few. In addition, byproducts of unsafe production processes dumped into the environment are poisoning the Earth's skin and enter our own.

One way to reduce environmental damage is by identifying which people need to stay away from specific exposures, which is something I do in holistic dermatology. The problem is that many of these exposures are widespread (such as in the atmosphere), or invisible, or both. Even if we could identify which people need to avoid a particular product, most products would be very difficult to avoid in today's world.

Many industries cater to our tastes, producing items that are harmful and even addictive when used in large quantities. Cigarettes, alcohol, sugar products, and even fried foods are in that category. Industry has even admitted to designing their products to have the most addictive quality possible, as in "foods" such as potato chips.

The combination of catering to our tastes and enticing our addition is not only a means to produce profit and create a driving force for commerce; for corporations with stockholders, it is a fiduciary responsibility. This means that they are *legally obligated* to their stockholders to produce a financial profit at the end of the year, even if it has hidden but serious health costs subsequently for the consumers and the world at large. I call the illness that emerges from the combination of addictive consumption "corporate irresponsibility and greed," and a legal structure that, in effect, supports all of this, a "social disease." Our society needs some big healing at many levels to heal the skin of the Earth, and improve our own skin.

The Broader Solution

There are very few people who would want to go back to the times before we had large corporations to bring us the production, technology, and advancement that is such an important part of our housing, food, transportation, communication, recreation, and medical care. There are many enlightened corporations that take on global health responsibility as a heartfelt obligation and not just a publicity issue or a way to avoid governmental sanctions and lawsuits. That these corporations are aware of the need to get on board with the "Green Revolution" is evident in full page ads showing how they are taking steps to save the planet. Social pressure, commercial value of a better image, and legal pressures all play a role. The problem is that there are many bad actors mixed in with those implementing change for the better. Rather than sanction, I believe that these companies need help in improving their products or in reducing the damage that is spewed from their production process. Some companies, such as some in the candy industry, need help in revisioning their products and mission, so that, for example, healthier treats are available to fill a nutritional void rather than to just appease hunger and taste craving.

Straggling and struggling industries need the big medicine of a new kind of team approach to deal with the social disease they are part of. One of the resources we have is the great number of highly trained graduate students who cannot get jobs. We need to put together scientists, engineers, industrialists, and lawmakers to find solutions to helping make production processes, products, and the use of those products healthier for our skin, our bodies, and for the skin of the Earth. We need to focus our resources on prevention at the source of the problems, rather than focusing on repair and sanctions and regulation, which should be a last resort.

What about products that are inherently dangerous or commonly used addictively and result in the advent of disease? I truly believe that if we perceive the problem, we can recognize the solutions. But we need clarity and we need transparency. I don't believe people should be prohibited from most activities that harm no one but themselves. On the other hand, I don't believe that everyone should have to pay to take care of the health of someone who chronically abuses substances that we know cause harm. So, for example, taxes on cigarettes should be earmarked and rigorously funneled to take care of the emphysema, heart disease, lung cancer, and other problems that befall smokers. Those taxes should not go to fix roads, make up deficits, or line the pockets of politicians. There should be a clear stream of that money going to the health care of the people who damaged their health by any known product, and the industry should pay a portion as well. It's just a matter of basic responsibility. The consumer and industry should have freedom, but *finance* the likely extra healthcare cost that is a consequence of their consumption.

The Individual's Solution

Making healthy choices in your home and work environment is a crucial step to healthy body and skin. For example, having a moldy house or carpets that de-gas aldehydes can aggravate allergic conditions of the skin. As you come to know your sensitivities, you need to make choices that will support the health of your skin. If you have pale skin and a history of melanoma in the family, you need to limit your sun exposure. You need to consider not only your sun protection methods, but where you live, your outdoor activities, and when you do them. If there are hormone-related cancers in your family, reading labels on cosmetics and anything you apply to your skin is important to avoid chemicals that may interfere with hormone metabolism. Everyone should read labels on food and on products that will be applied to the skin to verify that there is nothing to which they are allergic. For staying healthy, making the best choices in your exposures is the most sensible approach.

Are Comfort Foods Really Comforting?

Avoid eating to calm your emotions. The phrase "comfort foods" tells it all. It outlines the concept that we are actually eating to *comfort ourselves.* We're not even eating for taste, hunger, or nutrition. We're eating to distract ourselves from or cope with unpleasant emotions. Moving away from this kind of eating requires not only resolve, but also a truly supportive environment and a commitment to do what it takes to heal your inner issues.

Every culture has evolved food customs that teach balance, and unfortunately, also patterns of misuse of substances taken into the body, as well. Teaching appropriate use of substances (alcohol, narcotics, sugar consumption, etc.) has not been tackled effectively by most cultures, and seems completely lost in a world of addictions, improper and inappropriate use of food, and all types of narcotic substances. Alcohol is a major challenge in this category, so it is very refreshing to see the beer and liquor industries creating ads urging responsible use of their products.

Another way to make a difference in the bigger picture is to vote. You have at least three kinds of votes. You can vote at the cash register when you choose the healthiest food or cosmetics for yourself. You vote at the polls when you choose the leaders who care about your health or the laws that concern the environment that affects your health. You vote online when you give feedback or pass the word around to lawmakers or industry leaders about what you feel they are doing that is especially good or bad for health. Online campaigns are especially effective in empowering individuals to get their voices heard.

We've got to fix problems and clean up the show. A healthier and happier skin of the earth would lead to better health and healthier skin for all of us. The savings from a cleaner environment would help pay for companies to clean up their products and reduce toxins. Perhaps someday we will place more value on safe products and food than on abundance of adult and kid toys. The big question is whether we are really going to make significant changes in that direction, or continue to just move our mouths about health for everyone. We need to decide if we want to pour a fortune into healthcare, when good preventive steps could allow the current health care system to do a better job for more people for less money with the existing resources.

That is my vision of how our skin could change and improve by modifying the skin of the earth. I hope to plant the seeds of ideas that spread across the waters and fly on the wings of electronic communication so that more and more people find creative solutions to these looming problems. From my experience on an individual level, I know that the changes will take real commitment and not always be easy, but that the results will be beyond our greatest expectations.

Summary

The positive side of this story is that we, as individuals and as a species, have it in our power to improve our skin and our individual and global health by improving environmental conditions in our home, community, and planet. Real environmental consciousness is spreading throughout the planet. Just imagine: we can actually reduce illness and decrease health costs by cleaning up our environment. We have the ability to go through more of our life with health, vigor, and vitality. It is likely that hundreds of millions of people, if not billions, really prefer to not get sick from the unhealthy aspects of our environment.

Part 2

PREPARING FOR YOUR HOLISTIC EXPERIENCE

CHAPTER 18

SEVEN STEPS TO HEAL YOUR SKIN

When I first started to write this book, several people suggested I write it in the popular "how-to" style and call it "Seven Steps to Heal Your Skin." I tried to do it that way, but soon found that I had difficulty squeezing everything I wanted to say into that format. In fact, there are seven steps (see below), but they can only be implemented after you have some understanding of where your problems begin and how they might manifest themselves as problems on your skin. I believe that the complexity of information that's available is so great that having a simple cookbook of steps on how to heal a particular problem is virtually useless until you understand all the relevant factors that are involved and all the ways that you can view that information.

I've spent the first two-thirds of this book giving you a perspective that you can use to begin to understand what's going on with your skin and your body. Now that you have that perspective, you can start to make the changes necessary to clear your skin and inflammatory problems. The exercises that follow this chapter are designed to give you a running start on making these changes as easily as possible and with the least amount of resistance.

First you need to know that your efforts will pay off—you can get better. Then you need to gather information that both you and your health practitioners need to know as you go through the healing process. Finally and perhaps most important, I've offered suggestions on how to deal with some the personal challenges that you may face during your journey and ways to overcome them. Overcoming those challenges will have benefits in many other areas of your life, just as clearing up the skin problems from the inside will have benefits in many other areas of your health.

You may not need to do all the exercises that follow; you may already have sufficient commitment, willpower, and organization to make the necessary changes. For others, this guide may help in what seems to be an overwhelming task.

These exercises are the best way to start your journey towards better health and healthier skin. In this last section of the book, I'm asking you to do some work. You've read the book and obtained the information you need; now is the time for you to begin the three "takes" and seven steps:

Three Takes

1. Take stock.

2. Take help.

3. Take action.

Seven Steps

1. Get a diagnosis.

2. Write your medical history.

3. Educate yourself about the various aspects of your condition and its causes, or find a practitioner or coordinate a team who can help.

4. Identify likely underlying causes.

5. Correct the underlying causes.

6. Take the most natural or safest steps to relieve symptoms and appearance of your skin.

7. Commit to the process and stay with it.

Seven Steps Expanded

1. **Get a diagnosis.** If you have insurance coverage, or can afford to pay out-of-pocket, it is usually best to see a dermatologist or other physician familiar with disorders of the skin. A Western medical diagnosis is a good starting point, as it brings together much information about the spectrum of causes, underlying mechanisms of disease, risks of not treating, and likely ways to treat the condition. However, Western medicine may not be sufficient to explore all the causes that

can be helped by other healing perspectives. Once you have a diagnosis of a condition such as eczema that involves inflammation, it is time to look deeper for the causes of your inflammation. Other diagnoses may emerge if you explore functional, Chinese, or Ayurvedic medicine, or if you consult a homeopathic practitioner.

Sometimes, the diagnosis of the condition may appear obvious. Sometimes, an apparently obvious condition such as acne may actually be gram negative (bacterial) folliculitis or Candida folliculitis resulting from previous antibiotic treatment, and a culture by an astute dermatologist will be necessary to make that distinction.

From the perspective of the three takes, take stock; examine and list all the conditions or health impairments you have. Consider both those you have grown accustomed to, and those which are newly manifesting (for example, you have begun to notice pain in a few joints in your fingers a few times a week when awakening, or your nose was stuffy in the previous spring for several days when the pollen came out). Whether you have a diagnosis, or just a description of the issue, add it to your list. Then you can rate the severity, frequency, and duration of the symptom. You can also relate it to the cause you suspect is most likely (see Chapter 21, "Writing Your Patient History").

2. **Write your patient history.** The more you understand about the different perspectives and healing systems that may apply, the better your history will be. For example, when you read this book and understand the factors that lead to yeast overgrowth and leaky gut, you will remember events that have occurred that suggest whether or not that is an issue for you. The more your doctor understands, the more fruitful the application of that information is to your improvement. Many doctors are trained to examine, diagnose, and then prescribe the regimen of medication that treats the condition best. That may work well when, for example, a staph infection is treated with an antibiotic and there is no underlying issue that would make it return. But when there is an unidentified reason that a chronic rash keeps returning, it is time to investigate deeper. Some dermatologists are experts at identifying the allergens that cause contact dermatitis, by appearance pattern, history, and patch testing. However, many do not have the interest, time, or training to work with food allergy from a Functional Medicine perspective.

See the chapters on "Writing your Patient History" and "Your Wellness Evaluation."

3. **Educate yourself about the various aspects of your condition and its causes, or find a practitioner or coordinate a team who can help.** Reading this book will help you understand much more about inflammation of the skin, how it is related to what enters your body, and how the a variety of factors combine to make you better or worse There are some people who read medical and scientific literature and become highly self-educated so that they can make better-informed decisions. This is not practical for most people, so I have put together a section on how to build a team who can help. See the chapter "Putting Your Team Together."

4. **Identify likely underlying causes.** This requires correlating the preceding events with the findings on physical, laboratory, and other sources of information. All this information is then viewed and interpreted using a combination of perspectives from the healing systems that either you or your practitioner are familiar with.

   As you make your timeline or list of aggravations of your condition and preceding events, you will find that you will add specific relevant details as you increase your understanding of the condition and the mechanism of its cause. This information will be helpful to you and to your practitioner(s) in developing more certainty about the array of causes involved. The material in this book will help you see the interactive causal factors that I have come to understand in my decades of clinical care and research.

5. **Correct the underlying causes.** These various steps are discussed throughout the book.

   a. Improve gut flora.

   b. Improve digestion.

   c. Improve liver function.

   d. Fix leaky gut and leaky skin.

   e. Remove possible and likely environmental triggers: food, cosmetics, and topical applications, home and work exposures.

   f. Enhance removal of aggravators from your system, detox and aid your body's enzymatic machinery that breaks down and expels toxic materials.

g. When the benefits of resolving the internal causes become visible, or if you need external treatment ASAP, begin using topical treatment.

h. Commit to doing what is required to improve your condition and its causes.

i. Work on the emotional, psychological, and spiritual issues underlying your problem.

6. **Take the most natural or safest steps to relieve symptoms and appearance of your skin.** There is a series of natural steps to be taken that are discussed in this book. If, for example, an infection is present that does not respond to herbal or other more natural treatments, it makes sense within an integrative approach to advance to an antibiotic to prevent damage or danger. If the infection or inflammation is particularly severe or threatening, medical and even surgical care may be needed on an emergency basis, bypassing completely the natural treatments or using them, if appropriate, as ancillary help. In most instances, one has the choice to proceed with natural remedies or transfer to a more potent medical therapy. You may need someone knowledgeable in both conventional and alternative treatment to help you weigh these choices to avoid unnecessary harm.

7. **Commit to the process and stay with it.** Settle into a lifestyle that allows a shift in your condition. If the condition of your skin and your health cannot sustain the lifestyle and work demands you have, you have to make choices. Keep peeling off the layers of cause as they emerge and take steps to clear them. When you stop filling yourself with various sugary and processed foods, for instance, you may discover that those foods effectively suppressed unpleasant emotions; you will now have to deal with these emotions so that you can move forward.

Be persistent and patient. This can be a challenge. Sometimes, just taking a step such as avoiding sugar or gluten can tremendously improve an inflamed skin condition. In other cases, you may be pushing the edge of scientific research and understanding to determine how all the factors in your life and your genetics have influenced your skin condition.

You reached the point of having a persistent condition because of a series of exposures and habits that interacted negatively with your genetic YOU, and led you into a downward spiral, compromising all of your backup systems. Backup systems include a healthy intestinal flora, which like a healthy lawn, covers and keeps the weeds away. An intact intestinal digestive system converts foods to safe molecules, and an intact intestinal barrier prevents problem molecules from escaping into the blood supply and lymphatics. A healthy liver is able to filter out and break down problem molecules that do escape. Healthy immune system function includes the ability to suppress reactions against self that lead to excessive inflammation. Healthy adrenal function allows you to secrete not only adrenalin to deal with periodic stress, but the ability to secrete cortisone to calm down small inflammations that are not beneficial to the body as a whole.

Getting "un-sick" means unwinding that downward spiral, restoring the backup systems' ability to cope with a little stress, and allowing the systems to avoid and transform the memories, either emotional or immunological, that allow tiny triggers to initiate disproportionate reactions.

If the cause is harsh emotional memories, and you are strong enough, there are therapies that allow you to go through the pain of experiencing them, and then let them go. For some, such memories can persist for a lifetime unless the harm is forgiven. You must be a patient and earnest seeker to change the effect of memories that have been with you for decades. Some people even find that they must go beyond psychological and emotional therapies to a spiritual solution to find solace.

Summary

As you begin to correct underlying conditions, the overwhelming pressure is lifted from these backup systems, and they begin to function appropriately to resolve problems at the organ, tissue, cellular, and molecular levels. If damage accumulated over decades, resolution may require years. Proper diet can help; incorporating support with herbs and supplements will speed the repair of accumulated damage.

CHAPTER 19

YOU CAN GET BETTER

Heal Your Skin for Good

When we're born, we arrive on the planet with a clean slate. We're aware, we're curious, we're playful, and we're physically healthy. Our bodies and minds heal quickly. When a crawling baby bumps his head, his bruise heals in a few days. Colds and flu may come on strong, but pass through the system after a few days, and children are back to climbing trees, playing tag, seeing animals in the clouds, and giggling at being tickled. But through the course of life, this malleability and simplicity of body and mind begins to fade. Growing up in this society, having to fit in and make a living often means accumulating environmental toxins, absorbing emotional trauma, and sidestepping our truth. Our true nature can become buried in a sea of compromises. And without a routine practice of returning to our true nature, we find that the periodic itch, the sniffly nose one Monday, and the stiff shoulder after work last week slowly become a way of life.

How many chronic "way of life" problems have you accumulated with your skin and your overall health? Has uncontrollable acne made it embarrassing to walk into a room where other people have gathered? Has unending dry skin or an itchy rash made it impossible to concentrate at work or to wear clothes appropriate to the season? Has a continual craving for sugar made you spacey and overweight? Have you considered how they hamper your happiness or even make it difficult to get through the day? Have you tried repeatedly in the past to find a solution and it just hasn't worked? Are you fed up enough with a problem to find a way to finally resolve it? How much does your skin condition have to cost you in missed opportunities to participate in life before you invest the effort and money into changing the situation?

Can you imagine a life free from skin rashes, chronic itching, or tiredness? What would that kind of healthiness make possible in your life? I have been in practice for more than thirty years. I have accepted more and more patients who present successively more challenging, chronic conditions. They have seen doctor after doctor without finding relief, and have eventually shown up at my door.

I first obtain a very thorough, complete history of their condition. I consider myself a medical detective, examining each piece of evidence, researching each chemical pathway, and interviewing all the "witnesses." After working with many patients over the years, I have learned something amazing: you can get better.

Most patients I have worked with who have been diligent, forthright, and dedicated to finding and treating the underlying physical, mental, and emotional causes of their condition have experienced a beautiful transformation in one or more areas of their lives.

In these chapters I have included brief examples of people have made such transformations in their lives.

Back to the Source

Medicine has made significant leaps forward, riding on the rapid advances of discoveries in the various medical sciences such as biochemistry and genetics. Diseases were named and pharmacological treatments were developed to stop the manifestations of those diseases, sometimes killing the organisms that caused them, and at other times just stopping the inflammation causing the itch. Many people have been saved from trauma, infections, and acute medical diseases using this model. It's been so effective that we condescendingly view other healing systems throughout the world as quaint tribal approximations of real *scientific* medicine.

The same is true in the field of dermatology. However, moving from an era of trial and error with various potions and lotions to the use of scientifically-based treatments proven to treat various diseases, we have forgotten about the uniqueness of the individual patient in the narrow bottom line of improving the disease right now. In treating chronic conditions, too often the same medicine is used again and again, sometimes with loss of potency, creating the need for stronger medications the next time. Repeated use and stronger meds sometimes lead to unwanted side effects from the drug, such as thinning of the skin from steroid use. Or there may be persistent problems because the underlying disorder, for instance an allergy, deficiency, chemical toxicity, or hidden infection, continues, burning a hole in one's vitality.

tagged.

It's no wonder that people have been looking to alternative, holistic, Complementary and Alternative Medicine (CAM), natural, herbal, Chinese, Ayurvedic, and homeopathic worlds for ways to supplement or even replace conventional medicine and dermatologic techniques. I have been successfully applying alternative methods to the care of my patients with skin conditions for over 30 years. This book summarizes what I have learned over that period of time, and delivers a working plan to gain control of skin or other inflammatory issues.

You Can Get Better

If there is any moral to the tale of modern medicine, it is that treatment is available for even the most dire health conditions. From the tale of alternative healing, we learn that people can recover from all sorts of conditions that even conventional medicine cannot cure. Woven together, these two tales can create a tapestry of hope for potentially healing your skin or any other problem, should you grasp the appropriate information.

I wrote this book as a blueprint to broaden your understanding of the complex path to recovery from skin conditions and similar chronic conditions involving excessive inflammation, as well as to help you identify the many doctors, teachers, treatments, and transformations you may need along your path. My hope is that you have looked at it as an exciting journey of self-discovery, on which you have seen things you haven't seen before, felt things you haven't felt, and come to know parts of yourself you might not have met had you been "well." You can look at it as an opportunity to reach a level of balance and harmony with a depth of wellness and energy you have not previously known.

This does not mean that you can automatically solve the illness you are concerned about, but rather, that you have the *capability* to solve it and other problems you may suffer from if you have the drive, willingness, resources, and skilled guidance to do so.

Your journey may seem like a winding, unknown, jungle of a path but when you reach your goal, you will see in retrospect that the road you took was the straightest, clearest one that would bring you to success.

Guidance

Some people can actually take command of this journey, making the right choices at every fork in the road, independently. They can use this book to gather the right information and act upon it. I believe that these people are in the minority, but this book will be a helpful map for their journey.

Most patients, who have a difficult skin problem or other chronic disease and have sought medical help in the past to no avail, will need at least some guidance. They will also need some of the inner guidance demonstrated by individuals who can make this journey alone, because they are likely to hear differing opinions from different doctors, therapists, healers, friends, and relatives. One must be aligned with one's own greater good and desire for wellness, and not be derailed by self-destructive drives; only in this way will they hear clearly which suggestions are in their best interest, and which ones are issued to achieve control of their allegiance.

I do believe that skilled professional guidance is necessary. This may include a dermatologist or other appropriate specialist to diagnose the problem, from a Western, scientific medical point of view. Dermatologists gain great knowledge (and often some wisdom as well) from the years of training and practice that focus on disorders of the skin. You should avail yourself of their expertise, if only to be sure that your self-diagnosis has not missed some other disorder. It might be one that you have not considered: one which could respond to a very different treatment or one that needs more urgent care. An alternative practitioner may have some safer techniques to offer, but first you have to know what the disorder is, and that is best diagnosed by a physician. Unless there is financial hardship, it would be foolish not to take advantage of this diagnostic availability, especially because this is the most likely consultation and treatment to be covered under insurance.

You should also be educated by this specialist in the various treatments that are available, whether or not you choose to follow that path at the present moment. The knowledge will provide a platform of information regarding the steps that may be necessary, the procedures that are available if necessary, and the intensity of treatment that will be needed to resolve your condition. This information, in turn, will provide you a better idea of the effort you may need to put forth to transform your illness. For instance, if you are diagnosed with moderate to severe plaque psoriasis, and the suggestion is that you take one of the new "biologics" that selectively suppresses the immune system, you know you have a lot of serious work to do. When you hear that the drug costs twenty thousand dollars per year, plus doctor visits and lab tests, and engenders a risk of contracting tuberculosis, lymphoma, or a degenerative viral brain disease (along with the possibility of not even improving your psoriasis), you have an even better idea of the challenge it will be to clear your psoriasis without such drugs. In a case such as this, you must be tolerant of a lack of *instant* success; you must be prepared to try multiple methods and to incorporate some of the safer, time-tested dermatologic techniques such as tar and light treatment in an integrative approach, to reach a degree of improvement such that natural sun exposure in short-sleeved summer clothes feels comfortable to you and perpetuates the improvement of your condition.

Unless your more mainstream dermatologist has strayed from the beaten path (such as I and a few others have done), you will want to find an alternative practitioner who uses nutrition, herbs, and additional healing disciplines to bring you back to balance, and help you with your underlying problems which led to your illness.

If there are psychological or emotional issues that play a role in the vicious cycle of your illness, you will probably need some sort of counselor or psychologist to guide you to their release.

If you are wandering, lost in patterns that are years old, or even generations old, or if the road to recovery through any perspective seems unworkable, you may need Higher Guidance to find your way. Know that a path is always open to you, one that does not necessarily appear through your rational mind; a path you can see clearly only through your heart.

Learning can be done through books, informational websites, information groups by disease or disorder (for example, groups that avoid gluten) and professionally sponsored websites. You will have to evaluate the quality of the information by measuring it against other sources you know to be valuable. In later additions of this book, I will include a section at the end of the book listing resources for further reading.

Three levels of healing:

1. Soothe the problem: calm it down, reduce the inflammation, infection, and manifestations.

2. Clear the underlying issues that interfere with the normal physiology: this includes improving digestion, removing sources of allergy, and restoration of hormonal and physiologic balance.

3. Clear the mental, emotional and spiritual issues leading to the underlying imbalances and patterns that instigated the disorder.

Problems on your skin offer a direct signal and opportunity to explore the underlying issues at the core of your being. At their best, they can be a signal to you and to others that you need to go within and explore the depths of your imbalances. After all, an outbreak of acne is literally "staring you in the face" when you get up and look in the mirror. At the first level, you take and apply medicines or herbs to calm it down. Reaching deeper, you heal your dietary indiscretions, and the digestive and hormonal imbalances which are contributing. At the deepest level, you heal the silent, often subconscious, inner scream that only becomes quiet when you have finished the entire carton of ice cream, or whatever it is that you need to suppress uncomfortable emotions. Often you must look to Spirit for the strength to reach beyond what is rationally possible for you to attain. It is this spectrum of the third or deepest level of healing by which your skin problem offers direct access to healing your life and the lives of those around you. In the best possible light, you may see your problem as a unique reminder and opportunity to heal the deepest part of your being.

Rather than curse that pimple or rash, gather your inner strength and welcome the challenge to come through the process of healing at a healthier and more peaceful level. You may not even imagine the aspects of your life that will benefit from this healing, but you will watch them unfold along your journey.

You Have the Touch

The first touch of the skin of our fingers to the fingers of that special someone sends energy throughout both entire beings. Our skin is the connector, the transducer of this emotional explosion, like the needle in the groove of the record, connected to a thousand-watt sound system. The ridges in our skin, the ones that make our fingerprints, are alive with an assortment of nerve endings to transmit the kind of sensation that is occurring. Tiny sweat pores keep the right amount of moisture in the skin, determining how it will slide against another surface. And all the time we have signals traveling from our skin to our brain, tuning our motions, emotions, hormones, and even our genetic expression. Wow!

Seen in this way, our skin is not just another organ, but the living continuation of our life force itself. We damage our skin with sunburns, thorn-bushes, detergents, and chemicals, and it keeps coming back again and again. What we see when we view our skin is the product of a series of transformations of living cells to form a thin protective barrier that is constantly renewing itself, but is no longer made of live cells at its outermost layer.

When we see another person, we view their skin as it glides over their fat, muscles, and bones. Many of our conscious and unconscious reactions are based on what we see in their skin. We immediately judge age from the way someone's skin looks. A quick glance at sallow skin tells us that a person is sedentary or sickly. We often react even before we are aware of the judgments we have made.

Problems inside us may manifest as changes in our skin. Looking for what our skin is telling us about what is happening within us has become my passion. Examining both what occurs on the inside as well as the outside is what I utilize to understand why a skin condition erupts.

Summary

This book was written to illustrate that there is another way to heal your skin besides conventional medical therapy. Natural treatments can re-balance the body rather than block the mechanisms of disease and inflammation. For some people, that means there is a choice of either natural or conventional methods to heal their skin. For most, it offers a spectrum of treatments that can be combined, when chosen wisely, to give the most appropriate combination of conventional and natural methods for clearing up their skin problem. By placing an emphasis on the scientific rationale for various methods of addressing food allergy, gut flora, and digestion to clear skin inflammation, this dermatologist-written book places the natural techniques within a solid context. Presenting the integrative experience to you should provide you with confidence in choosing integrative techniques, which should make it easier to implement the changes in your life that are necessary to explore a safer way to improve your skin, and the health of your body.

CHAPTER 20
YOUR WELLNESS EVALUATION

The chart on the following pages will help you keep a running assessment of how well you are doing. It can give you a perspective on whether or not the treatment you are using is taking you in the right direction, especially if the changes are slow and incremental, and you forget how the symptoms were before you began the program. There are a number of different scales for evaluating how you are doing for comparison after treatment. Some standardized tests have the advantage of being validated by multiple studies. What I suggest here has the advantage of being more appropriately oriented to both your skin and your psyche, and to the underlying organ systems that seem to be involved. A good program should improve mental and emotional issues while improving digestion and the skin. Record notes on any life events that seriously impact your mental and emotional state that might set back your overall improvement.

	Pre-Program	One week	One month	Three months
Rash				
Describe area of coverage on your body				
Duration of appearance				
Degree of severity of rash cycles				
How much does the itching bother you				
Allergies				
Nasal drip and itchy eyes				
Sneezing				
Cough				
Digestion				
Abdominal bloating				
Pain				
Nausea and/or vomiting				
Diarrhea and/or constipation				
Gas or discomfort after eating				
Tired after meals				
Energy Level				
Always tired, never enough energy				
Not sleeping well				
Energy level remains constant throughout the day and after work				
Not enough energy to work a 40 hour week				

	Pre-Program	One week	One month	Three months
Other Physical				
Headaches				
Muscle aches				
Joint pains				
Emotional State				
Contentment				
Joy				
Sense of humor				
Love and gratitude				
Frustration				
Sadness/grief				
Fear				
Anger				
Mood swings				
Mental State				
Mental fogginess				
Clear-headedness				
Agile and coordinated				
Quick reaction time				
Obsession and/or compulsion				
Craving				
Peace of mind/peace				
Forgetfulness				
Anxiousness				

CHAPTER 21

WRITING YOUR PATIENT HISTORY

There have been many times in my practice when a patient with a rash or recurring skin condition comes to see me and is at a loss to explain why this outbreak has occurred. When I ask them to tell me everything that occurred before they broke out again, they say, "I don't know. I'm eating all the same things I usually eat. There's nothing different." Only when I dig and probe and ask pointed questions do they realize they have done something different or eaten something unusual or added new products to their daily routine. Unfortunately, many doctors don't have the time to sit with their patients and ask probing questions.

This is one of the key factors in the kind of medicine I practice—to understand what's taking place "underneath." The more I can help patients understand what it is I'm trying to do, the easier it will be for them to provide relevant information to me and to any other of their health professionals. The better the history the patient can compile, the better their outcome is likely to be.

The inflammation that causes skin rashes comes from something or somewhere, even if it is difficult to identify what that something is. The entire premise of this book is that we can find something about the cause and do something to reduce or eliminate it. If there was some factor causing the problem, it was usually occurring prior to problem becoming evident. To find the possible cause or causes, it is critical that you take some time to answer the questions below. As you learn more about your condition from your practitioner, this book, or other sources, your answers will become more relevant. For example, if your symptoms worsened on April 15th, you might remember that it occurred on the day you paid your income taxes. If that was a non-stressful occurrence, it might be irrelevant information. But if the issues regarding paying taxes stressed you out for days or weeks, and you couldn't eat right or get enough sleep while trying to complete the forms and pay the money you owed, this might be very relevant to the onset of your condition.

Here are the three main questions you should be asking:

- What occurred in the days and weeks before your problem first appeared?

- When did your problem get worse or get bad enough to seek care?

- What occurred in the days, weeks, and months preceding *the aggravation of* your problem?

This is crucial information for the practitioner who is seeking to find the underlying cause of your skin condition and improve it by correcting that cause or causes. It is the start of further inquiry, examination, and testing to elucidate additional answers, and treatment for the probable underlying causes. The practitioner who is simply treating symptoms may disregard this information and proceed to use the medication that is most appropriate to suppress the condition they see.

One method of maintaining your patient history is to record your outbreaks, treatments, reactions, and improvements on a timeline. What information should you collect, and how should you structure it in a way that will enable a physician help you ferret out the triggers for your skin (or other) disorder? This section will help you expand your thinking to construct a better history.

What Is So Important About Your Story?

When a patient comes to see me about a skin condition, the first thing I ask them to do is to write Their Story, and bring it to our first meeting. How do you write "your story"? This is really important because it is something that you can develop over time and refer to or have your practitioner refer to as appropriate when you are ill. The careful telling of Your Story can reveal what is causing your condition, how your body works, what specifically is wrong, and even hint at what parts of your genetic code are "open" and producing protein products or signals. The new field of "epigenetics" is the study of what genes are turned on (what part of your genetic code is being read to produce proteins) in your body and how their products are modified as opposed to simply what genes you have inherited. Various conditions you experience, and the compensations your body makes to stay in some sort of balance, all involve accessing the proper aspects of your genetic code. You can think of our chromosomes that contain our genetic information as a wall full of working reference books. When you select a cookbook from that shelf, and open it to a specific page and choose a recipe to make a dish, you can imagine that you are doing something similar to what your cells do when they choose to access and read sections of your genetic code. They do not prepare all the recipes in the book all the time. The concept of epigenetics also involves a further step. For various reasons, our cells modify messages made by the genetic code and their products, just as we might decide to modify a specific recipe in the book. When you arrive with a particular skin disease, you have accumulated many activated genes that are reacting to, controlled by, or compensating for the allergic, infectious, or toxic substances involved in your condition.

Knowing what has been taking place in terms of consumed foods, environmental exposures, and emotional experiences that might have modified how your physiology altered normal activities such as digestion, all provide hints about what might be triggering your rash. Like the shadows on the wall in Plato's cave, you cannot see the actor; but you learn much about him from the outline of the moving shadow. Likewise, the experienced practitioner sees trends and patterns according to the systems they understand, and can probe with further questions and testing to confirm or reject the suspicions they have regarding what is causing your skin issue and how to correct it.

You may have thought about your skin condition and what was taking place near the time it started, and can't make any sense of it. You are eating the same basic diet and avoiding the same foods. Nothing seems to be changed in your food or work or life pattern. How can anyone else figure out the solution? The skilled physician brings various forms of understanding to the situation, asks further questions, and then sees how different pieces of information fit together into a pattern suggesting a reason for the outbreaks. They do this according to all the systems they understand. In my case, I consider nutrition, functional medicine, herbal medicine, immune system relationships, industrial chemistry, environmental chemistry, and to some extent Chinese energetics and homeopathic relationships. Just like the mechanic who hears the story about your car, listens to it, and then uses his or her specialized knowledge and experience to interpret the information, I interpret the story of the body. When you hear a rattle in your engine, telling your mechanic the whole story sometimes helps so that he or she can fix the car without harming it or the people in it. The same goes for the body.

Early in my clinical training at Bellevue Hospital I had a supervising physician who made a startling remark: "If I had to share a workup with a subordinate, and *had* to choose between taking a patient's history and doing a physical exam, I'd take their history and let the subordinate do the physical." Keep in mind that we were untrained and inexperienced at the time. We were just learning how to listen to hearts and lungs, and the information obtained from the physical exam seemed to be of paramount value! So why would he make this statement? In dermatology, seeing and touching the skin problem is necessary for making a diagnosis. I often get crucial information from photos of a patient's rash at its worst, and how it progressed over time, via a quick tour on their cell phone. This was not usually possible before the modern world of digital information and smart phones. Nevertheless, much experience in the world of complementary medicine was required for me to appreciate that for understanding how to treat the underlying cause, an accurate and complete history *is* the most crucial part of the data.

I can remember on past occasions asking a patient what was taking place and getting the reply, "You're the doctor; you tell me." I'm quite capable of making a conventional diagnosis by examining a patient's skin condition. And I can often guess something about the possible causes from the combination of the visual exam and the superficial information I get from observing the individual and asking what kind of work they do. But actually finding the cause requires the patient to pull out the nuggets of information that will make my understanding more accurate. The certificate that hangs on my wall says Dermatologist, not psychic. I need the cooperation of my patient to probe the causes just as much as I need his cooperation to make changes and eliminate the factors that are causing the skin condition. This kind of medicine requires a team effort to succeed, with the patient being an active member of the team.

Remember that recording what you ate just before a breakout, for example, might have more meaning to the skilled practitioner than it does for you. Some items might be suspect by themselves. Other exposures might build and build until your immune system finally explodes and over-reacts. Some culprits may cause outbreaks because of their similarity to other allergens or because one modifies the response to another. Instead of dismissing information, making assumptions, and coming to your own conclusions, record the data, keep searching your mind for more details, and let the practitioner decide.

As you understand more about the nature of the mechanisms underlying disease, you will be able to select more pertinent aspects of your history and present them to your doctor. For example, when you understand which reactions are caused by a "delayed hypersensitivity," you will look at what took place 48 hours prior to such outbreaks, knowing that some outbreaks take at least that long to appear. When you realize that some exposures "open the gate" to let other exposures cause inflammation, you will see that food exposures in a particular sequence can cause many more problems than single exposures alone. While you understand that some specific foods, such as crabs or nuts, might trigger a reaction, you may not realize that something you eat all the time might accumulate in your system or create a hidden food allergy. That's why I ask you to compile and write down all the information, even if it seems mundane. After all, if you could see all the patterns already, you would probably have corrected the problem yourself.

Telling Your Story

There are two purposes for taking some time to compile your history. First, it will prompt you to think about and remember the events and sequences of events that occurred near the time that your skin condition began or worsened. Second, it will help you begin to place those events into a time sequence, so that we both will have a better idea of what came first and the order in which they happened. This information provides an idea of what may have caused a reaction to occur. I start with suppositions, and then ask more questions to explore them further.

To tell your story, start with a large piece of paper (or initiate a document on your computer). Draw a big horizontal line across the paper. Add the date and details of your outbreak somewhere on the line. Then, think of times before that one when you had any kind of small similar outbreak. Record their dates and details on the time line as well. Were there any holidays, important events, or travels that you can remember before or after the outbreak? Also list those in place. Often such events, and whether the skin condition existed before or after them, help pinpoint the event in time.

What other big changes, illnesses, operations, or injuries have occurred in your life? Go back to the timeline where you listed your outbreaks, and fill in the times of these events as well as anything else you can think of in terms of medications taken, foods eaten, unusual exposures, allergic reactions, moving, or whatever else you can think of that might have occurred just prior to your outbreak. Keep inserting events and exposures that took place before and after your eruption time as you remember them. However you do it, you will be compiling a sequential timeline of what occurred before and after your skin condition started.

Many physicians have been taught to dismiss this sort of information, since it may be irrelevant to making a conventional clinical diagnosis. If a doctor is looking for the cause of the condition, rather than just the diagnosis, this information becomes very important. Most physicians don't have the time to pursue this kind of questioning in a busy, insurance-based practice. Furthermore, since other forms of knowledge are required to understand nutritional and environmental causes, they often do not have the training to analyze the information. Although they may hear something that would cause them to direct a patient to a specialist, they often don't know when a holistic or complementary physician could best treat a patient.

Let me give an example: When a patient's problem comes after a trip out of the country, I inquire whether there was any diarrhea after that visit. This could indicate a parasite or other intestinal infection, which could lead to bacterial changes influencing the immune system or to food allergies. If the problem occurs after a surgery, I inquire whether antibiotics were given, which could lead to yeast overgrowth in the intestines.

Another example is a musician I saw with a rash around her mouth. Her dermatologist treated her for a combination of the two likely conditions, contact dermatitis and perioral dermatitis, but the rash only got worse, becoming more red, uncomfortable, tight, and unsightly, even with makeup. I had her stop everything she was applying related to the rosin on her bow, as well as the other medications she was given. Only in my questioning at our second encounter, after she had improved dramatically, did I discover that she had had a severe reaction to some unknown sunscreen in the past. Knowing the likely chemical structure of the sunscreen, I realized that the sulfonamide-related medication she was prescribed for perioral dermatitis was probably a substantial contributor to the cause of her contact allergy. It was very similar chemically and allergy-wise to the sulfonamide-related sunscreen. In this case, a more complete history would have helped even if the understanding of the chemical relationships was absent.

I suggest that you put together your own history, especially if you have persistent skin problems. Even if you cannot see a relationship between events and outbreaks, you will have the information in place when you meet a doctor who can help you interpret it. And who knows, it could even be fun to look at the recent events in your life and draw connections and meanings you hadn't noticed before.

History of the Present Illness

You might want to create an outline that follows the more traditional intake histories that physicians use. That way, you will be able to present pertinent information to your physician in a way that he can easily digest and will give him more time to focus on the most important issues and possible causes of your condition.

When and how did it first appear? Remember events or holidays around that time to see if you can pinpoint the exact dates. Look at a calendar. Was there some activity you could not do because of the rash? When you have pinpointed the date, think of the events in the days, weeks, or month that preceded it. Was there any illness, new medication, food that made you sick? Just make lists without judgment. Most people have gone over this in their own mind searching for clues. In the process, they often have dismissed important information because it was something that happened regularly in the past without incident. Be complete, so that your holistic provider will have the information needed. Some conventional doctors may be able to work with this information and many not. But put it together anyway. Someone else will surely have more perspective than you do. If they are skilled in this work, they will be able to make all kinds of connections between what occurred before the rash appeared and the possible causes of the rash. They will question you further to test the validity of the various possible causes, generated by your experience and the nature of your condition.

If you are fluent with a computer, list the times of outbreaks on a word processor document. Then go back and add information pertaining to what occurred before each outbreak, what treatments were used, and how well they seemed to work. List the treatments that worked or did not. What other changes in diet or lifestyle might have made a difference?

Related History

You might also want to note other skin conditions you may have had; other allergies, to what and when they were triggered; and anything else that seems related to your condition.

General History

You should also prepare a brief summary of any medical conditions you have had (not necessarily skin-related), when they occurred, how they were treated, and how well the treatment worked. List accidents and surgeries, and medications you have taken in the past and you are taking now.

List other kinds of treatments you have had, including supplements, and how effective they have been.

Summary

Some people choose to make one chronology of all of their histories, both skin and general, and this works well. Remember that a good practitioner must envision the whole picture to have a chance of seeing how important trends interact and are related. Most dermatologists, like other specialists, really focus on just the condition in question and don't place much emphasis on everything else taking place. The kinds of treatments that calm down skin disorders don't require this expanded view, and their patient load would not permit obtaining this level of detail. If the condition is self-limited, and clears after one or two treatments, the limited approach is a more efficient method of care. But if the condition does not clear or persists and becomes chronic, identifying the cause becomes more important. I want to emphasize that my colleagues in Dermatology do try to look for the specific cause, especially in the case of conditions such as contact dermatitis or infectious skin conditions. And most dermatologists do understand the chemical relationships among various products that cause allergy in the skin. They usually do not have time to probe beyond the most targeted questions. Unless the solution involves elimination of gluten or a contact allergen, they just stop short when lifestyle and diet play a role; they usually have neither the belief, the time, nor the knowledge of how to clear the condition with natural techniques.

Exercise: Outbreak/Exposure Record

If you are a very organized person, with a problem you really want to solve and the time and motivation to keep a diary, you may keep an exposure and condition diary. Many people are not so thorough. If you do not keep such a diary, there is another way to help a skilled doctor help you: when an outbreak occurs you can write it down everything you ate and what else was taking place during the 48 hours prior to the skin eruption.

There are now some modern tools that can help you keep track of your foods and other potential environmental irritants in connection with your outbreaks and other symptoms, including apps for your smart phone, such as my Symptoms, Food Diary, Food Allergy Detective, and many others.

Some people keep their food diary and symptoms list on the spreadsheet, and still other people just keep it in a journal.

When your rash breaks out or becomes aggravated, sit down and write down everything you ate and were exposed to on the day that you broke out and the two days previous to that day. Do this instead of wasting any energy fretting. You will never remember as well what you ate if you wait a week or more until you see the doctor, so do write it down as soon as you can. You may begin to see yourself some relationships between exposure and outbreak. A well-trained physician should be able to see relationships that you have not seen, and help you identify the culprits causing your condition.

As you probably can see, keeping a diary like this has the potential to help you identify what is contributing to a variety of conditions besides your skin condition.

The essential elements of a progress diary to determine what is most likely causing your problem are as follows:

Exposures and Treatment Program   Changes in your Condition

Exposures and Treatment Program	Changes in your Condition
Percent of the time you followed diet:	Condition of your rash
Did you cheat on the diet?	Skin worse after cheats?
Foods you ate:	Deterioration? New lesions?
Supplements taken or left out:	Improvement?
Home or office painted, sprayed for pests? Major stress or upset?	Status of allergies
Medications you took:	Other health conditions
Other exposures?	Improvement in energy? Digestion? Other?
Anything seem to make things worse?	Any problems, aggravations or side effects?
How did you know it was worse?	Initial "cleansing" or die-off reaction?
Which supplements or dietary restrictions seemed to help especially?	

"Other" exposures could include anything unusual, either in the realm of physical or emotional, even if you do not register the presence of that factor. For instance, loss of a job will surely have emotional consequences, even if you do not feel that right away. Lack of sleep, or conflict at work or in a relationship can change how your body systems perform. Other examples of exposures which could really affect you could also include recent indoor painting or spraying for pests. In the second column, "other health conditions" might include headaches or return of other symptoms that you have had in the past apart from the rash or skin condition you are working specifically to clear presently. Brief but diligent notes on your observations need only take a minute or two several times throughout the day.

A Typical Work Sheet Might Look Like This:

Exposure	Condition/Symptom and Percent of change	Time, Date of Exposure	Time, Date of Symptom
Breakfast: bagel, cheese, coffee	slight itch on elbows after breakfast	8 am, Tuesday March 2	three hours after
Lunch: salad with chicken	rash getting redder on left arm	12:30 pm	immediately after lunch
Smelled air freshener spray in bathroom at work	felt dizzy	2:00 pm	one hour after
Dinner: potato, broccoli, steak	rash seemed to improve 25%	7:00 pm	over the course of the day

How a doctor hears your history depends on their depth and areas of understanding. For instance, a dermatologist skilled in industrial contact sensitivity will hear your work history and have a good idea what substances to test and what questions to ask to determine if various exposures and contacts are related to the same allergic chemical. A knowledgeable physician who seeks the cause of your problem and reads a carefully remembered history of how your condition started, and what events, illnesses, stresses, and chemical exposures preceded that condition, is better equipped to reach a diagnosis of the causal chain of events.

CHAPTER 22

WHAT REALLY BUGS YOU?

For some people, skin problems are an expression of the pain and conflict and other emotional issues that are taking place internally at any given time (as discussed in Chapter 5). Answering these questions may help you become aware that you are suffering emotionally and that this may be contributing to your skin condition. Then you need to ask yourself if you can handle these issues on your own or if you need to seek professional help. Ask yourself these questions to get at the emotional issues that get under your skin (ouch!).

For some people, this is no small challenge. For others, just becoming clear and aware can free them relatively quickly.

Often, the skin speaks information we cannot. Make a list of things that have "gotten under your skin" and really bug you. Put them in categories:

- Things that bug me and I speak about/act on directly:

- Things that bug me and I speak to other people about them, but I take no action:

- Things that bug me and I speak to other people about them, but no one seems to hear me:

- Things that bug me and I don't speak about; I only feel them or think about them within myself:

- Things that bug me and I don't even let myself know how I really feel about them (this is the most difficult and perhaps most valuable question):

- Things that bug me but there is really nothing I can do about them, so why get more upset trying or even thinking about trying to change them:

Write the answers to these questions in a notebook, and add to them as more answers percolate to the surface of your thinking. You may find that there are sensible steps to take to release much of the pain you carry or experience over and over again. Make notes on how to release and get beyond each of the things that bug you. Often, you first have to identify them and then let yourself experience and release the pain that is involved. Sometimes, just identifying the assumption or belief you hold regarding why something *should* bother you brings instant relief. Other times, simple appreciation and forgiveness can give release. If you have deep emotional wounds or are emotionally fragile, you may need professional help with this step. Remember that even the sandpaper that abrades your mind is smooth on the other side. Turn it over.

CHAPTER 23
WHAT GETS IN THE WAY?

Are there emotional issues that are emerging in my behavior towards my skin? Should I be dealing with those issues? Are social pressures interfering with my ability to determine if a particular method will be beneficial, and if so, do I need to face the question: Is getting better more important than the social pressures I'm feeling? Whether it's an alternative program or a physician's prescription, at some point you have to decide if you are willing to follow it well enough to ascertain if it's the right direction.

Ask yourself if these are the factors that interfere with your healing and self-care:

- I don't want to give up the foods I like to eat.

- I can't hang out with my friends if I have to eat so differently.

- I hate to take pills. I can't swallow them; they make me sick; they're too much bother, I always forget to take them.

- I have created a response that's turned into a habit that's turned into an addiction.

- I really think that somewhere out there is some special pill that will make this all go away without any side effects or effort on my part.

- Am I capable of making a commitment?

If I were to imagine my skin problem benefitting me in some way, what way would that be?

• Me

1. Scratching and picking gives me pleasure, *takes my mind off more disturbing issues.*

2. It is safer to feel less attractive.

3. I want to let the world know how angry, depressed, etc., I am, but cannot express myself openly.

4. It hides the real me.

5. It hides the deep shame, pain, and other emotions I feel.

6. It lets me be left alone by others.

7. It lets me be alone in my own private world.

• Family, friends, spouse

1. They don't believe that I am sick.

2. They think I'm too sick and keep me feeling that way.

3. They don't think that I need to do the diet, etc., as suggested.

4. They believe that I am on the wrong path, that I should follow their way, another way.

5. They think that I should lighten up, forget the restrictions, take a break, and have a good time.

If you wish to improve your health with a natural method and find yourself blocked, take the time to think about each question honestly. Write down the answers in a notebook. With a vibrant picture clearly in mind of the healthy you who has successfully overcome your condition, start finding answers for each question. Do not be misled by the wish that one magic pill will make you all better with no other effort or cost.

You may find that the answers to some of the questions above reveal bigger questions (and opportunities for growth), some of which will require a new path or the help of a therapist.

CHAPTER 24
PUTTING YOUR TEAM TOGETHER

Each time that I work with a new patient, I like to put a team together. We call it, "Team You." Team Joe, Team Sarah, Team Fred—you get the idea. For some people, I am all they need for a team because I am both holistic and a dermatologist. There are very few dermatologists who practice the way I do; so, from a practical standpoint, you will need to build your own team. And many of the people who come to see me already have some sort of team assembled, including practitioners with whom they feel comfortable and who can address their various emotional and physical issues in a manner that suits them. This may include therapists, energy healers, acupuncturists, general MDs, dermatologists on their insurance plans, nutritionists, and more. Often this group provides more complete support for an individual who is struggling with a number of interactive issues.

On occasion, however, I find myself in a situation with a patient's other healers act as if one of them is guarding the ball in a tough game of pick-up basketball. One of the practitioners wants to take control, and will criticize treatments, undermine suggestions, maintain control of the patient, or be sure that their remedies are utilized while they are kept secret from the doctor (me). That is a bad situation for your chosen primary practitioner, and an even worse one for you. I remember a case of a young woman with a severe yeast infection complicated by infected contact dermatitis of the vaginal area that continued unendingly. I determined that she was sensitive to certain oils used as fragrances (essential oils), but much questioning and two more visits were required to discover that another practitioner was giving the patient these very oils in his "special" nutritional food. For that reason, it's important that you share whatever treatments you are undergoing and any medications you are taking with everyone who is on your team.

It is important for just one practitioner to be the team leader, and make his decisions on the basis of the results that occur. Some people come to me because they have not gotten effective help so far. If the previous healer is making therapeutic changes at the same time, it becomes impossible for the new practitioner to know which treatments are working and which are aggravating the situation. This can also be true for the patient who goes to a series of different healers before they even have time to try what the first one suggested. The sense of urgency is understandable, and the desire to do everything possible is laudable; but the patient has to either be highly intuitive, or more skilled than any of his healers to put together a sensible program from a series of often-conflicting suggestions. And they lose the opportunity to see if a stepwise program can make a difference, since they never give anyone a chance beyond the first or second visit.

You want someone who understands both worlds—if they have great techniques in Reiki or Acupuncture, but they have no idea of the biology of melanoma, they can do you great harm. It is therefore important that you choose a healer to master your care who has knowledge of both traditional dermatology and alternative practices, and then put together a team, that can truly work with each other, or at least synergistically, for your benefit. Think of it as remodeling a house; you would need to choose a general contractor to be in charge of coordinating the other various skilled craftsmen to make it all work.

Each person's team will look different, depending on their condition, location, resources, and needs. But I will outline here what composes some various teams, as well as the responsibilities of each team member.

The Top Five Questions to Ask Yourself When Assembling Team You

Ultimately, the answers to these questions will be up to you, but here are some places to start:

1. Who is calling the shots, to coordinate things? Will he or she be the primary healthcare practitioner regarding this, and my current issues?

2. Who else will I see to support the direction of my primary practitioner, or to take care of other issues that the primary practitioner agrees are unrelated and need specialized care?

3. How much will I see each practitioner?

4. Is it likely that the practitioners will communicate with each other? In

person, if they work in the same office? By phone? You know how hard it is to reach your doctor or how hard it is for them to reach you. It can take weeks of phone tag to make contact between busy practitioners. Our HIPAA laws make it technically illegal to discuss your case using unencrypted email, and getting two people on the same encrypted system is no easy matter.

5. How can I benefit the most from meetings and heal the fastest?

The Top Five Questions to Ask Prospective Practitioners When Interviewing Them for Team You

First, remember that each practitioner has progressed along their own path to doing the medical discipline that they do. Although there may be many approaches they share with you, it is pretty unlikely that they will share all the same strengths, opinions, and beliefs that you have. They may be very open-minded, but they are not you.

1. Does the practitioner you choose to be in charge have expertise in the areas of the body within which your condition lies, or in the condition itself?

2. Are they on the same page as you regarding the methods of treatment you prefer to try first?

3. Do they have a clear endpoint at which they would refer you to a more conventional or more powerful treatment? Can they explain what your options would be?

4. Can the additional members of your therapeutic team support your main practitioner, not making therapeutic changes that will confuse the situation or undermine the overall direction?

5. How long would they expect you to see results (minimum and maximum) so that you know how long their therapy needs for a fair trial?

Each Team Member's Primary Responsibilities:

You: Deciding who to work with, and taking responsibility for your health; following the guidelines agreed upon by you and your team; getting help when something is difficult or overwhelming, finding the support you need; asking the questions you have, bringing with you to visits and meetings your complete and organized history and information; being open, honest, and willing to see and feel what you haven't seen and felt before. If you do not follow the suggested program, no one will ever know if could have potentially benefited you. If you make up your own rules, you may be missing the main points of your treatment, requiring repeated visits until you understand and follow the plan you are given to evaluate whether or not it improves your condition.

Your Primary Physician/Holistic Healer: Must have a great understanding of both you and the type of issue you have, and whose methods you feel comfortable utilizing. This person should have a perspective that will move you along to improvement of both your presenting and underlying issues.

Alternative Specialist: If there is a major issue that is blocking your progress, you need someone on your team who can help you overcome it. For instance, if there are emotional issues that drive you to eating patterns that aggravate your problem, you need effective help dealing with those issues. If there is a highly specific organ system that is part of your general health, you may need a specialist in that field to at least monitor its activity, if not actually help with the treatment. For example, a reproductive endocrinologist might be needed for severe hormonal imbalances. This is not the time for experimenting and trying every modality you have not yet tried. There will be time to try other modalities when you either find indications that they may improve your results, or when you have exhausted the benefits from your primary holistic approach.

Western Specialist: Should be current with the latest diagnostic and therapeutic options from the standpoint of scientific medicine, and be able to provide a clear diagnosis or list of possible diagnoses, from a disease standpoint. They understand the science behind your disorder, and can rationally evaluate some of what you are choosing for your direction to improvement. You may not choose to do what is recommended, but you can learn the options, and find out at what point the specialist believes irreparable harm will be done if you do not use the suggested treatment. They should discuss with you any controversy regarding their recommendation, even if considered the standard of care. For example, high risk is associated with failure to have a lesion highly suspicious for melanoma properly excised, but additionally having a regional lymph node removed has been the subject of some controversy. You should preferably choose someone who is at least open to discussing your choice of path if it is not the treatment they recommend. However, if they are not supportive of an alternative option, do consider that they may view the option as dangerous to your health from a Western medicine perspective, and therefore, are reacting from concern, not closed-mindedness. You may need to provide evidence that you do not hold them responsible for the choices you make, even by offering to sign an agreement acknowledging your refusal to follow the physician's recommendations and stating that you understand the possible dire consequences; in this way, your choices do not burden the doctor with a possible legal threat because he did not follow standard of practice guidelines.

Therapist/Healer: Provides individual support and tracking; really helps you explore yourself and your perceived limitations; sees you as a whole, healthy being; helps you overcome issues that keep you from following a program or diet; for example, a program that removes the emotional support you derived from eating particular foods.

Group: Provides weekly and daily emotional, psychological, and spiritual networking in the form of meetings, phone calls, or emails. People experiencing similar challenges can help you feel less alone and more connected, can share success stories and hope, and can provide connections to physicians and healers who they have found helpful.

Extras: Depending on the issues that become apparent as you seek transformation to a healthier trajectory, and the specific outer and inner changes you will need to make as you move along that path, you may need additional help. You may find that you or someone close to you can actually take on these roles, if you cannot afford to hire the help. Let me stimulate your imagination for other possible ways to fast-track your way to optimum health in Lifestyles of the Emotionally Rich and Famously Whole. Here are some suggestions that can help you to actually create community with your healing. There are many ways to achieve the same goals. Sometimes all it takes to garner support for your goal is to ask. Here are some suggestions:

Personal Trainer: Can help you focus and shape your physical endurance, flexibility, and sense of well-being. Even taking classes at a local gym can be very helpful in these areas.

Life Coach/ health coach: Keeps you on the path of prioritizing the actions you need to take, and being accountable for accomplishing them. A group or team can help in this regard, as well. If you can't afford a life coach, you may be able to find a life-coach-in-training who wants to practice or is looking to build up his or her clientele. You can also try trading time with a friend; you can each check in every day to monitor each other's goals, to ask how things are going, describe what you have done well where you'd like to improve. A health coach who supports you in following your main practitioner can be valuable. A health coach who steers you away from the direction of your main practitioner can disable your program, unless you truly believe that the coach should be the person to manage your care.

Personal Chef: Prepares healthy meals within the context of the dietary eliminations and supplementations you are following, and makes them enjoyable to eat. If this option is not feasible, you can cut out recipes and hire a friend's son or daughter to help you prepare a host of tasty, wholesome meals for the week; enroll in cooking classes or read about cooking the kind of diet that would make you the healthiest you can be.

Spiritual Guide: For those who see no rational way to accomplish the changes required for better health, given their condition, circumstances, failed repeated attempts to change how they act, and the "baggage" they carry, a spiritual solution can often offer hope for change. This guidance could be in the form of an individual (e.g., a minister, priest or rabbi), a spiritual group, or even a 12-step group. Always be clear about the ongoing cost of the transaction.

Exercise: Professional List

Make a list of professionals you'd like to consider working with and inquire each of them regarding availability. Be ready to provide a short summary of your condition and your patient history. They will have their own resources to assemble a team, but you should have a team of people in mind.

- main care provider/coordinator

- specialist in your problem area

- therapist

- healer

- support group

Choosing Modalities that are Right for You

There are a number of important real life considerations in choosing what modalities to use. They fall into the following categories:

Effectiveness and appropriateness: Just as in conventional medicine, where we are accustomed to visiting a specialist for the eyes when we have vision problems, there are Integrative physicians who have expertise in particular organ systems (such as the skin).

Safety: Many natural treatments have far greater margins of safety than conventional treatments, but this must be weighed against the more rapid and certain efficacy of conventional care. This knowledge must be included in the benefit and risk evaluation for any healing modality.

Feasibility and Flexibility: There are real considerations about costs of treatment, including what you can afford comfortably, and which aspects may be covered by insurance. These are strong influences on what path an individual may choose. Also of importance are the types of clinics or healing therapists available locally, versus one's ability to travel for treatment. Because lifestyle change and giving up favorite foods is often required for natural treatment, the ability to change, whether via willpower or spiritual strength, is often critical for this work to be successful. Using new systems of healing depend not only on how much you can learn and understand, but on how well you can stretch your belief systems.

Most people start with what fits into their comfort zone within the considerations above. Will their insurance company cover the visit, is the practitioner they need in the same town, do they believe in the new method suggested, are they willing and able to give up favorite foods, drinks, chemical exposures where they live or work, and so forth. If they can do all of that, they proceed with a modality recommended. If not, they have to carefully weigh the alternatives, and look at the costs/rewards of the proposed modality. They will have to consider whether they can move beyond what is comfortable to do. They may have to travel, spend money which was earmarked for other purposes, suspend disbelief about an unfamiliar healing system, choose the modality for which there is a good practitioner nearby, or seek help making life-style changes they have struggled to make, unsuccessfully, for years.

Writing Exercise: Support

- A holistic program will involve changes in many aspects of your life. When you understand what is involved, you need to enlist those who care about you to support your efforts, perhaps despite their own beliefs, to ensure you have a good chance of success. Journal about what changes you anticipate needing to make, and the blocks to success that you and other people close to you will construct.

- What shifts do you need to make, and how can you make them?

- What issues or beliefs are in the way?

- What do you have to do to ask for help; or can you secure support through demonstrating that your program is helping you?

- Who do you need to follow a healthier program?

Summary

Organize your answers to the questions posed, to create an outline of the plan to address your condition, and begin to implement it. Keep track of what you have done, how you are progressing, and what else needs to be accomplished.

CHAPTER 25

VISUALIZE YOUR FUTURE SELF

This exercise will help you develop a goal. It's similar to a chosen destination when you're sailing. Instead of going around in circles, you select a point that you're aiming for, which helps you organize how you steer and you trim your sails. Visualizing will bring your previous exercises in line with the goal. If you don't have yourself organized, you will bounce in and out of your commitment. The visualization exercise is designed to help you organize your direction, your consistency, and provide you with the power to make all this happen. There is tremendous value in visualizing what you're trying to create.

No house is ever built without a vision of the final structure. Getting your own "house" in order requires that you visualize the image of that order.

Exercise: Visualize Your Future Self

While sitting straight up in a chair with your feet on the ground, close your eyes and take some deep breaths. Relax and feel yourself grounded in your chair, and feel your breath, picturing it moving through your body to your feet.

Now begin to imagine your future self, healed. How will you know that you are healed? What will you feel, look, be like? What will the world feel, look, taste like?

What do you see is possible now that you are free from this persistent condition? Let it be playful and fun! Who would you be? What could you do that you are not comfortable doing now? Feel yourself being that free person.

Draw a picture, write a poem, or just write about your vision. Write about your commitment to your health from this place of freedom.

When you are ready, share your vision with someone who you trust and who supports you, and make a commitment to yourself, in their presence, that was established in your vision. Agree to check in with this person on a regular basis regarding your commitment.

When you are firm in that vision, decide if that is what you want to achieve, with no holds barred, and if you are willing to do whatever it takes to get there. Are you willing to give up favorite foods and make changes in your habits? Are you willing to organize your life to make these changes? Are you ready to experience greater energy, better digestion, reduction of allergy symptoms, and a likely pathway toward a healthier, longer life? If so, you should be able to overcome obstacles to follow this program, and lean on those you trust to help guide you.

Conclusion

You have just read a blueprint for integrative treatment of the skin starting with the use of safer, less invasive, more natural remedies. The information is based on my initial and ongoing training as a dermatologist, my learning and research in Immunology, my study of other methods of healing, and my experience during decades of practice. I hope that you will now entertain the premise that inflammatory skin diseases have a cause that can be known with a degree of certainty, and hence be corrected. Much of that correction is by eliminating or remedying environmental aggravators that precede the onset of the condition, using natural remedies. The largest source of foreign material in the body is the gut, so the treatment plan needs to emphasize treating the digestive tract.

It is hoped that some basic understanding will help you better interpret your past and your unique responses to various aggravators as well as beneficial treatments. Digestive function, immune recognition and cross reactivity are all concepts you should better understand for interpretation of your health-related experiences.

I pass along this information to my readers to help them find answers to their skin issues. For the physicians and scientists, I hope that these ideas will at least pose questions they may not have asked, by offering a new conceptual framework for understanding the causes of skin disorders. These are not final answers; I hope to continue my exploration to refine further the understanding of inflammation and skin disease.

ACKNOWLEDGEMENTS

First, I would like to acknowledge my daughter Alicia Dattner for the tremendous amount of help she gave to this project and her humor in meeting challenges that arose. I would like to thank my rewriter, Sharyn Kolberg, for her patient and skillful editing, and my illustrator Ronnie Ray Mendez for his insightful and humorous illustrations. Nancy Cleary, of Wyatt-MacKenzie Publishing has done a wonderful job assembling the book and moving it into print, and Karen Kibler, a microbiologist herself, was patient and efficient in the skillful copy-editing on the book. This book could not have existed without what I learned from all my teachers, colleagues, and patients, who are too numerous to mention by name. A short list of medical mentors includes Doctors Barry R Bloom, Eli Seifter, Lloyd Old, Boyce Bennett, Mark Hardy, Arthur Fox, Frank Pass, Michael Fischer, Arye Rubenstein, Felix Rapaport, George Degnan, Peter Pugliese, and William R Levis.

NYU School of Medicine had a spectacular group of immunologists during my years of medical school training including Doctors Kurt and Rochelle Hirschhorn, Fritz Bach, Baruj Benacerraf (later won Nobel prize), Chandler A. Stetson, Bill Paul, and Bert Gesner.

My Integrative medicine education advanced, in the days before this was popular, via members and guests of the AIMS group including Doctors Leo Galland, Michael Schachter, Steve and Ken Bock, Stephan Rechtschaffen, and Dan Kinderleher. Doctors Robert O Becker, Jeff Bland, Jonathan Wright, Alan Gaby, are just a few of the guest lecturers at AIMS and elsewhere who have added to my knowledge.

Applied Kinesiology training came through Doctors Sandy McClanahan, David Leaf, George Goodhardt, and especially, William Maykel.

Herbal training came from attending herb conferences and from a variety of teachers including David Winston, David Hoffman, and Michael Tiera.

I credit my psychological/emotional/spiritual learning to both my challenges and blessings, and to those who offered perspective: Murshid Samuel L. Lewis ("Sufi Sam"), Pir Vilayat Inayat Khan, Shlomo Carlebach, Swami Satchitananda, Zalman Schachter, Victoria DeMasi, and Brian Ahern.

Insight, suggestions, and criticism were provided by a number of author friends including Barbara Wexler, Douglas Gasner, Frank Asch, Goldie Milgram, and Michael Samuels, MD. Ray Chambers supplied encouragement and support toward completing this book project. Words do not suffice to express the appreciation for my wife, Shohama Wiener, whose patience, support, editing, and encouragement during the process of creating this book allowed it to come to completion.

APPENDIX

Resources for Healthcare Professionals:

We hope that this book opens communication with the rest of the world about the methods discussed. We would like to invite the following interactions as described in this section.

Please follow carefully the suggested protocol for each type of interaction described below so that we can properly read and respond to yours. Below are a list of the various inquiry categories and how they should best be addressed and written:

To Medical Schools and Medical Research Institutions

Please contact me to arrange for consultation, projects, workshops, lectures, ongoing advisory programs, or establishing Integrative Dermatology at your institution.

To the pharmaceutical industry

Fear not: success with Integrative Medicine methods listed in this book requires self-motivation, diet, and lifestyle change for success, *combined* with knowledge of appropriately-timed use of both natural substances and medications. At this time, the majority of the population will not find it convenient to follow the regimens required, and will still need pharmaceutical products to control their illness, so that your current pipelines and market approach will still be in demand and vital to our healthcare system. Many of the people who do seek to follow the methods listed in this book would not use pharmaceuticals for skin problems either because of their firm personal preferences, or because they tend to have adverse reactions to everything from ordinary fragrances to common medications such as aspirin. You are best to have this population self-select away from potent medications rather than tarnish your product's image with a high percentage of adverse drug reactions. Undoubtedly these individuals have a much higher than normal likelihood of SNPs that make it difficult to metabolize drugs.

Despite the tremendous success of the pharmaceutical industry, many patients are plagued by the increasing complexity of their illnesses. There is a huge frontier opening for assessment of disease, prevention, greater choice in therapies, and modification of the conditions leading to illness, with the potential for pharmaceutical companies to actually serve as key players. The knowledge base is evolving with various healing systems outside Western medicine, from basic science discoveries, to physicians who are incorporating this knowledge into their practices. Integrative physicians have a population of patients with complex diseases, which make their offices a living laboratory, providing hints on dealing effectively with the plethora of complex and unsolvable disease situations that are becoming more and more common. Encouraging this living laboratory to thrive opens opportunities for everyone to mine this knowledge base and direct its evolution into an effective total diagnostic and therapeutic approach to the specific patient with their physician.

Possibilities include everything from improving selection criteria for drug use, to maximizing benefits and minimizing side effects, and could be accomplished using techniques from the "alternative" medicine world. Proving algorithms with sophisticated laboratory assays and then correlating less costly existing integrative screening techniques is just one way that integrative medicine could help improve choice of pharmaceuticals for best results. As I see it, the value of drugs *as part of that process* increases greatly when targeted toward the individual with an integrative approach. Companies that expand beyond the old model of drug for disease, and instead start measuring and incorporating data to guide physicians to tailor treatments, will develop a track record that will quickly put them ahead of the old model.

Preserving the multitude of approaches to healing allows this data mine to grow, so that new products can emerge. In the long run, suppressing integrative medicine is like slashing and burning trees in the Amazon, including the ones that help cure cancer—the fire warms you for a week, but the cure is lost forever.

Patients with complex issues such as autoimmune diseases related to chronic viruses, Lyme disease, etc., are sometimes better helped through different methods. The linear model of drug for disease is sometimes less effective than the patient-specific unraveling of causal factors in returning these patients back to productive lives.

Individual specificity in treating illness comes from, in part, our understanding of genetic and epigenetic individuality, as well as exposure history, and has been an important differentiation point, as well as marketing point for both natural products and pharmaceuticals. The pharmaceutical industry has the technical resources, funding, and sophistication to expand into the world of diagnostics, as it relates to discerning and suggesting targeting for the underlying causes of illness, perhaps better than any other industry.

Given the scale of need in the area of diagnostics, high-tech vetting of integrative diagnostic techniques could provide the public with feasibly priced data to help in the selection of both natural products and pharmaceuticals. Effectively screening out the majority of patients likely to have an adverse reaction could permit use of some medications otherwise excluded because of side effects. This could lead to a more effective, safer set of treatment options, a less expensive health bill, and healthier work force. There is room to invest in, and benefit from, a priority shift.

Furthermore, a more sophisticated evaluation system of individual variables that could be accomplished on a large scale, for minimal expense, would enable identification of those individuals destined to have adverse reactions to new drugs. The world of integrative medicine contains many low-cost systems of evaluation that could be vetted with scientific studies for screening; for example, greater risk of drug reaction or the most efficacious drug to use. Integrative diagnostics could also be used to choose supplements or other drugs that could overcome Single Nucleotide Polymorphisms (SNPs, single genetic mishaps), to prevent the abnormal metabolism of such drugs that lead to adverse or fatal reactions. Some of the new drugs that have been discarded, or will be, because of such adverse reactions, might still be usable with such laboratory discernment. The natural product world is a vital incubator for both such products and evaluative processes. Suppressing the natural product incubator would eliminate vast amounts of human experience-based knowledge that could otherwise take decades to evolve again. Natural methods should be viewed as a resource rather than a competition, to be mined as Sherlock Holmes used the "Baker Street Irregulars."

Natural methods could also be used to counter the many side effects that are endemic to a subset of the population who uses pharmaceuticals. Just one small example is the use of probiotics after antibiotic treatment. Integrative therapy expands on this. Protecting the gut mucosa with use of NSAIDS or protein pump inhibitors is another area where integrative methods can reduce clinical harm. We can help with these challenges, and numerous other instances to smooth out the overall therapeutic results of a combined approach.

It is crucial to remember that integrative methods are already being used to ameliorate the side effects of drugs. To squash public access to such natural treatments will not only destroy the incubator of such methodology, but also will raise the overall morbidity of drug treatment in the world today, and may make many pharmaceuticals no longer fit for the marketplace. Integrative physicians and teams like ours who use both pharmaceuticals and natural therapies can provide advice in adding value to application of pharmaceutical therapeutics in the evolving world of new possibilities and expectations.

To Neutraceutical Cosmetic and Cosmeceutical Industry Partners

We are interested in product development, refinement, and matching the right product with the right patient situation. Having dealt with industry offers during the past few decades, I am only interested in those who truly value my contribution so that I have a chance to build upon repeated successes to develop products in my own pipeline that will make a major impact on inflammatory disorders.

To readers with interesting experiences

If you wish, please share your experiences with skin improvements achieved as a result of reading this book, at **http://holisticdermatology.com**, using our contact form. In your email, be sure to give us permission to use your comments on our website. Unfortunately, we do not have the resources to give feedback, answer questions, or treat you on the basis of your comments (however, you can book a patient visit with Dr. Dattner on our website).

To those seeking Holistic Dermatology treatment or coaching

For people with mild to moderate acne who would like to begin making changes before one-to-one treatment with me, we are developing an online program that will be available through our website. For those who need more individual treatment, we can be contacted as below.

Our website is **www.holisticdermatology.com**, and you can contact us there to schedule Holistic Dermatology treatment or health coaching via online video. Please know that if you work with us, you will need to make diet changes that eliminate some of your favorite food items, and that you will need to take several supplements. We do not accept medical insurance. Patients pay out of pocket for treatment and supplements. Some of those expenses may be reimbursed if you have out-of-network coverage, and have met your deductible or have a flexible savings account for medical expenses. We hope that someday, the kind of in-depth care we give may be covered by insurance. It is ironic that some insurance companies will pay up to eighty percent of the nearly $300,000 per year it costs to treat advanced melanoma skin cancer with two new drugs, and up to $50,000 for new psoriasis drugs per year, but will not cover the relatively miniscule cost of treatments utilized by integrative physicians who save the system money in the long-term, by fixing underlying problems and, for example, returning patients with chronic fatigue to work, so that they can be productive and happy again.

To patients with "unsolvable" skin conditions, or other inflammatory illnesses that have persisted for years or decades, looking to "contract" a solution finally

In the academic world, developing solutions to complex health problems often requires many years of research by entire teams of physician scientists, sometimes extending through entire careers and consuming millions of dollars. Requirements for proof and the tangle of bureaucratic nightmares involved slow down this process tremendously.

For individual patients, in some cases, our team will have the ability to treat your health situation in a far timelier manner. If we have the specific skills and interest required for your needs, we can potentially create and oversee a program to guide you to a solution in a stepwise manner.

Please contact us through the query form on the website to arrange further consultation. Please note that we are not able to give medical advice on the basis of what you write alone.

Investors with similar values

We have projects in various stages of development that are ripe for investment potential, provided that the terms of the investment allow us to guide the project, and guide the subsequent projects in our pipeline.

To Dermatologists looking for training in this medical discipline or to partner in this work

We are in the process of developing a training program to guide and train dermatologists interested in Integrative Dermatology, and in learning to treat patients in an integrative and holistic fashion. A limited number of applicants will be accepted for this program, including one to work directly with Dr. Dattner. This program will evolve a network of practitioners able to handle disorders often in a safer and more effective manner than with conventional diagnostics and therapeutics alone.

For those dermatologists with extensive relevant basic science and/or integrative medical experience, there is potential room to learn, share knowledge, and invest in and become part of the core of the forefront of an exciting buildout of integrative and holistic dermatology and its science-based products. We want to broaden and deepen this methodology and to build it out as a sub-specialty of dermatology that interacts with other current methodologies to greatly enhance the overall effectiveness of dermatologic therapies as a whole. Contact me with your CV and interest via my website (**www.holisticdermatology.com**).

To my fellow physicians and dermatologists

From the perspective of current practice, the totality of the methods I am putting forth may seem completely foreign. Yet it is based on the immunology and science that underlies inflammation as the pathophysiologic mechanism causing the condition. A substantial portion of my understanding of these mechanisms came from my work on cellular immune cross-reactive recognition in the dermatology branch of the NCI in the late 1970s. I was examining patients for the cause of their cross-reactive stimulus for decades before this understanding became widespread at the turn of the century in 2000. Tools from the worlds of nutrition, herbal medicine, environmental medicine, Applied Kinesiology, Functional Medicine, Chinese Medicine, Aryuvedic Medicine, homeopathy, and emotional/spiritual healing have all added to my ability to reverse the stimuli for inflammation with a more natural approach.

This understanding has been productive in helping a large percentage of the patients who are willing to make the necessary changes in their diet, lifestyle, and supplement regimen. As it has developed, it has been clear to me that these mechanisms yield a better causal understanding of many skin conditions. I have published some of this information in peer-reviewed literature, and in Fitzpatrick's Dermatology. Many of the individual methods and concepts that I discuss have individually been used by or discussed by other dermatologists or reported in the peer-reviewed literature as *in vitro*, animal, or human studies. I know the preferred method is to justify such conclusions by journal reports, so I apologize to those who see me extending the nature of the mechanism of various dermatoses beyond what is currently documented in the literature as I include the mechanisms I see during the course of treating patients. I aim to get this information to the world expediently, and hope that funding for such confirming studies will follow, and that others will continue this work. I hope to follow this book with a text for dermatologists, and more case reports on my findings.

One reason that this type of approach has not yet become widespread is that extended time with the patient is required to explore the network of environmental causes, and determine diagnoses and treatments involving the digestive, immune, hepatic, hormonal, and emotional systems; a patient must be well-motivated to make dietary changes and be able to afford to take supplements. One impediment to patients' understanding of the complex conditions and treatments is that crucial information on biologically active ingredients is frequently hidden from proper labeling and disclosure. It is even more unfortunate that dermatologists cannot receive compensation from insurance companies to study the complex information involved, and to take the time to work with patients, when drugs used to treat the same condition are covered by insurance at a much higher cost.

I use my own "fuzzy logic" to integrate my understanding of the individual and the HLA-specific nature of cross-reactive stimulation of inflammation to explore hints that will identify a patient's trigger, both in the history of their onset and in the aggravation of their disease. I find that as I learn more about the web of factors leading to inflammation, I also hear more in the patient's history to guide my understanding of etiology and subsequent treatment.

I hope this book helps give you a perspective on another method to treat diseases of the skin and inflammation, for those patients who do not respond to other forms of therapy.

Government and private insurance companies

Returning ill people to healthy, happy, productive lives is a shared goal we all have. Let's benefit the health of our American population as efficiently as possible. Good public health planning and disease prevention requires stemming the tide of current environmental crises like oil spills, industrial pollution, and more, which accumulate and burst forth as disease when people are in the height of productivity, and affect entire generations ahead.

Another issue that affects public health is the favoring of the least-trained health practitioners, or for the least form of care, who end up diagnosing improperly or prescribing poor treatments, resulting in the risk of having to invest subsequent balloon payments for the problem in the future. Our system is already under strain. Let's instead pay now for doctors to properly identify patients' issues and gain control of their diseases. Let's instead motivate people and industry to offer healthier products, and reduce the toxin levels, because not doing this almost always costs us more in the long term. Let's set up legal structures that actually support the avenues of care that can potentially help patients, instead of so many of the current ones that impede care.

Let's consider compensating integrative physicians more money for the complex work they do, because it will cost less in the long run. The significant cost of new drugs is an indication and reflection of the magnitude of scientific power we can bring to treating diseases. If a drug costs $10,000 to use, and has significant potential side effects, this is an indication of the difficulty of treating the disease. This cost should help define the average cost of treating various simple and complex disorders, whether with pharmaceuticals or not. If integrative physicians can bring additional skills, time, and motivation to patients to treat for a lesser average cost, they should be properly compensated to reduce the cost to insurance companies from the savings obtained.

Let's not set up legal structures that foster or create illness, while at the same time touting the idea of health and healthcare for as many people as possible. For example, government subsidies to tobacco companies paved the way for millions of Americans to get cancer, and someone has to pay for their treatment. Today, we may no longer subsidize tobacco, but we permit toxic or carcinogenic levels of substances to enter our products and environment. We allow tanning booths to operate, which increase the likelihood of cancer, without targeted taxes to care for the increased level of melanoma they produce.

Both Integrative Medicine and good Conventional Medicine require detective work to find out what is aggravating a patient's condition. To yield the best health outcomes, our laws should improve, rather than obscure, the ability of both patients and physicians to know exactly what is in the products we eat and contact.

We have the information to make political decisions that help the health of our people and the environment that sustains us. We are at the edge of an era with vast new possibilities for maintaining and restoring health, with the awareness and merging of multiple healing systems with medicine. We have ever-enlarging scientific capability to refine our thinking, and discern new combinations of treatment that are most applicable to both the general and individual situation. Hopefully, healthcare will embrace the new options offered by Integrative Medicine, and cover the cost of that care when it is less costly than other options. With all of this, we have the opportunity to have a healthier, more productive, happier, population that will lead to more beautiful skin on people and on the face of our planet.

INDEX

CPSIA information can be obtained
at www.ICGtesting.com
Printed in the USA
FFOW04n1025220417
34735FF

9 781942 545163